STUDY GUIDE

ABNORMAL PSYCHOLOGY

STUDY GUIDE

PATTY ROSENBERGER
CORI ANN RAMÍREZ
Colorado State University

ABNORMAL PSYCHOLOGY

THOMAS F. OLTMANNS

ROBERT E. EMERY

PRENTICE HALL, *Englewood Cliffs, New Jersey 07632*

©1995 by PRENTICE-HALL, INC.
A Simon and Schuster Company
Englewood Cliffs, New Jersey 07632

10 9 8 7 6 5 4 3 2 1

ISBN 0-13-148792-2
Printed in the United States of America

Table of Contents

PREFACE

Your instructor has selected an excellent textbook on abnormal psychology. The material presented in your text emphasizes both the latest information on clinical disorders and the description of major research paradigms used in this area of study. We hope that you will enjoy learning about this fascinating area of psychology.

As you read through your textbook, note that all of the chapters are organized similarly. Every chapter begins with an overview of the types of disorders that will be introduced in that chapter. A description of the typical symptoms and associated features of the disorders is then presented, followed by a review of major classification issues, including current diagnostic criteria for each disorder. A discussion of epidemiological aspects of the disorders follows, focusing on incidence, prevalence, and gender and cross-cultural differences. Etiological factors that contribute to the development and manifestation of these disorders are then presented. Finally, treatment approaches to the disorders are discussed. Each chapter concludes with a chapter summary. Being aware of this broad organizational outline will help you organize and study the chapter material more efficiently.

Throughout the chapters, you will notice key terms that are bold-faced. The definitions of these terms are important for you to know. The terms are listed at the end of the chapter and in the glossary at the end of the book. There are additional important terms that are italicized but do not appear at the end of the chapter or in the glossary. Additionally, at the end of each chapter of your textbook, you will find a chapter summary. This summary is a detailed abstract of your chapter, and it will be helpful if you review each summary before working on the questions included in this study guide.

This study guide is organized to maximize your efficient review and comprehension of the material presented in your textbook. Each chapter begins with a **CHAPTER OUTLINE** that parallels the outline featured in your textbook. Studying this outline will help you organize your review of the material presented in your text. The **LEARNING OBJECTIVES** highlight specific ideas, concepts, and issues that you should understand. The **KEY TERMS AND CONCEPTS** list the bold-faced and italicized items included in your textbook for your review. **KEY NAMES** of people who have made important contributions to a particular area are also listed. It is important for you to be able to know these individuals and their particular contributions to the field. The **MATCHING** and **MULTIPLE CHOICE QUESTIONS** will help you determine your strengths and weaknesses regarding mastery of the material present in your text. Finally, answering the **BRIEF ESSAY QUESTIONS** will help you integrate information that has been presented throughout the chapter. In addition to answering these essay questions, it is important that you review the critical thinking questions that can be found at the end of each chapter in your text.

We hope that you will find this study guide to be a valuable resource for your work this semester. Reviewing all of the sections and completing all of the exercises for each chapter should be very helpful as you prepare for exams. Good luck and enjoy your course!

STUDY GUIDE

ABNORMAL PSYCHOLOGY

CHAPTER ONE
EXAMPLES AND DEFINITIONS OF ABNORMAL BEHAVIOR

CHAPTER OUTLINE

Abnormal Psychology: An Overview

Conceptualizing Psychopathology
    Case Study: Schizophrenia
        Associated Issues
            Defining Abnormal Behavior
            The Official American Psychiatric Association (APA) Definition
    Case Study: Eating Disorder
        Associated Issues
            Dimensions versus Categories
            Epidemiology

Causes of Abnormal Behavior
    Case Study: Substance Dependence (Alcoholism)
        Associated Issues
            Nature and Nurture
            Systems of Influence
    Case Study: Depression
        Associated Issues
            Biological Reductionism
            Cause and Change

Further Questions

Goals of this Book

Summary

LEARNING OBJECTIVES

After reviewing the material presented in this chapter, you should be able to:

*   know a basic definition of abnormal psychology

*   understand the scientist-practitioner model

*   consider the three primary criteria of abnormality (personal distress, statistical rarity, and maladaptiveness) in terms of their strengths and weaknesses

* distinguish the dimensional approach to abnormality from the categorical approach

* know the terms epidemiology, incidence, and prevalence

* describe the nature-nuture controversy in abnormal psychology and explain why it should not be a controversy since nature and nurture interact

* explain the meaning of the diathesis-stress model of abnormality

* compare the individual, social, and biological systems of influence

* define and understand the advantages and disadvantages of biological reductionism

* understand that changes due to a certain form of treatment do not prove causality

KEY TERMS AND CONCEPTS

Following is a list of key terms and concepts that are featured in the chapter and are important for you to know. Write out the definitions of each of these terms and check your answers with the definitions in the text.

Psychology
Psychological science
Abnormal psychology
Scientist-practitioner model
Clinical psychology
Psychiatry
Psychosis
Delusion
Hallucination
Disorganized speech/formal thought disorder
Psychopathology
Syndrome
Schizophrenia
Insight
Gender identity disorder
Phobias
Diagnostic and Statistical Manual of Mental Disorders
Premenstrual dysphoric disorder
Bulimia nervosa
Categorical approach
Dimensional approach

Quantitative
Qualitative
Threshold model
Epidemiology
Incidence
Prevalence
Etiology
Case study
Nature-nurture controversy
Diathesis/vulnerability
Stress
Diathesis-stress model
Biopsychosocial model
Psychopharmacology
Psychotherapy
Cognitive therapy
Biological reductionism
Descriptive psychopathology
Classification
Methodology
Treatment

KEY NAMES

The following individuals/cases have made important contributions to the material presented in the chapter. Write out the names of these individuals or the court cases presented and the theories, research, or treatment with which they are associated. Then check your answers with the information in your text.

Blue Shield of Virginia v. McCready
Wyatt v. Stickney
Jane Murphy

MATCHING QUESTIONS

Match the following terms and names with the definitions presented below. The answers can be found at the end of the chapter.

a. incidence
b. developmental psychology
c. nature
d. hallucination
e. etiology
f. psychiatry
g. epidemiology
h. prevalence
i. abnormal psychology
j. comparative psychology

k. clinical psychology
l. nurture
m. categorical approach
n. cognitive therapy
o. psychology
p. methodology
q. syndrome
r. case studies
s. delusion
t. dimensional approach

1) _____ the viewpoint that psychopathology is caused by genes, infectious diseases, physical injuries, or malfunctions by the brain or other parts of the nervous system

2) _____ the scientific study of behavior and mental processes

3) _____ formal description of the experiences of individuals who suffer from various types of psychopathology

4) _____ an idiosyncratic belief that is rigidly held in spite of its preposterous nature

5) _____ concerned with the application of psychological science to the assessment and treatment of mental disorders

6) _____ classifies behavior in terms of a continuum ranging from normal behavior to a dramatic extreme

7) _____ refers to the number of new cases of a disorder that appear in a population during a specific time period

8) _____ a perceptual experience in the absence of external stimulation

9) _____ the application of psychological science to the study of mental disorders

10) _____ a group of symptoms that appear together and are assumed to represent a specific type of disorder

11) _____ the branch of medicine that is concerned with the study and treatment of mental disorders

12) _____ formal procedures used by scientists to collect data in order to test hypotheses

13) _____ the scientific study of the frequency and distribution of disorders within a population

14) _____ traces the growth of factors such as cognitive abilities, emotional responses, and personality traits from infancy to old age

15) _____ viewpoint that experience is the central cause of abnormal behavior

16) _____ another word for describing causes of psychopathology

17) _____ classifies disorders in a dichotomous fashion

18) _____ refers to the total number of active cases, both old and new, that are present in a population during a specific time period

19) _____ helps patients identify and correct patterns of illogical thinking and maladaptive assumptions

20) _____ examines the same, or analogous, phenomena in other species, placing human behavior in an evolutionary perspective

MULTIPLE CHOICE QUESTIONS

The following multiple choice questions will test your comprehension of the material presented in the chapter. Circle the correct choice for each question in the section. Then compare your answers with those at the end of the chapter.

1) According to the DSM-IV, all of the following are examples of personality disorders EXCEPT:

    a. depressive personality disorder
    b. paranoid personality disorder
    c. borderline personality disorder
    d. antisocial personality disorder

2) A type of formal thought disorder, the prominent feature is severe disruptions of verbal communication.

    a. depression
    b. schizophrenia
    c. psychosis
    d. disorganized speech

3) This refers to a disease that was caused by a vitamin deficiency in people whose diets included relatively large quantities of unprocessed corn which induced psychotic symptoms that resembled those seen in schizophrenia.

    a. pequena
    b. pelo
    c. pellagra
    d. pesca

4) The assumption that biological explanations are more useful than psychological explanations because they deal with smaller units is called:

    a. biological perspective
    b. genetic predisposition
    c. biological reductionism
    d. medical model

5) In the United States, major depression affects:

    a. 1 in every 10 women
    b. 1 in every 20 women
    c. 1 in every 40 women
    d. 1 in every 50 women

6) This model combines the dimensional and categorical approaches to classification.

    a. threshold model
    b. scientist-practitioner model
    c. diathesis-stress model
    d. biopsychosocial model

7) When literally translated, the term "psychopathology" refers to:

    a. "deterioration of the psyche"
    b. "pathology of the mind"

c. "pathology of the psyche"
d. "deterioration of the mind"

8) An extreme, circumscribed fear of a given stimulus is called a:

a. psychotic reaction
b. fetish
c. delusion
d. phobia

9) A mental disorder is typically defined by:

a. one distinguishing symptom
b. statistical rarity
c. a set of characteristic features
d. the individual being out of contact with reality

10) These two disorders are much more common in women than they are in men.

a. alcoholism; antisocial personality disorder
b. anxiety disorders; depression
c. alcoholism; depression
d. anxiety disorders; antisocial personality disorder

11) One important point illustrated by the case of Gina King (depression) is that:

a. it is impossible to treat depression without medication
b. success of treatment does not prove the cause of the problem
c. depression only occurs as a result of situational variables
d. cognitive therapy is not sufficient for treating depression

12) Beth shows delusional thinking and hallucinations. Bob shows hallucinations and formal thought disorder. According to DSM-IV:

a. they could both be classified as schizophrenic
b. they would be given different diagnoses
c. they probably have different etiologies
d. they should get different treatments

13) All of the following are hypotheses of the etiology of abnormal behavior EXCEPT:

a. diathesis-stress model
b. biopsychosocial model
c. biological reductionism

　　　　d. scientist-practitioner model

14) The approach that defines psychopathology in terms of signs and symptoms rather than inferred causes is:

　　　　a. descriptive psychopathology
　　　　b. influential psychopathology
　　　　c. comparative psychopathology
　　　　d. experiential psychopathology

15) All of the following are ways in which case studies can be useful EXCEPT:

　　　　a. provide important insights about the nature of mental disorders
　　　　b. allow you to draw conclusions about a disorder from a single experience
　　　　c. aid a clinician in making hypotheses about a specific case
　　　　d. provide a rich clinical description which can be helpful in diagnosing
　　　　　 an individual

16) According to your text, almost _____ to _____ percent of bulimic patients are women.

　　　　a. 55; 60
　　　　b. 65; 70
　　　　c. 75; 80
　　　　d. 85; 90

17) _____ is a disorder that is first evident during childhood and adolescence.

　　　　a. dependent personality disorder
　　　　b. multiple personality disorder
　　　　c. conduct disorder
　　　　d. schizophrenia

18) These two disorders are much more common in men than they are in women.

　　　　a. alcoholism; antisocial personality disorder
　　　　b. anxiety disorders; depression
　　　　c. alcoholism; depression
　　　　d. anxiety disorders; antisocial personality disorder

19) All of the following could be considered psychotic symptoms EXCEPT:

　　　　a. delusions
　　　　b. hallucinations

c. disorganized speech

d. illusions

20) Eating disorders can be fatal if they are not properly treated because:

    a. there is a high suicide rate among people with eating disorders

    b. they affect so many vital organs of the body

    c. people with eating disorders are often unaware of the disorder and therefore are prone to developing additional disorders

    d. the majority of people with eating disorders do not view their behavior as problematic and therefore do not seek treatment

21) Blue Shield of Virginia v. McCready and Wyatt v. Stickney were two landmark court decisions in the early 1970s that:

    a. allowed licensed clinical psychologists and social workers to treat patients without the supervision of a psychiatrist

    b. allowed licensed clinical psychologists and social workers to prescribe medication to patients with the supervision of psychiatrist

    c. maintained that licensed clinical psychologists and social workers need to be under the supervision of a psychiatrist while treating patients

    d. allowed licensed clinical psychologists and social workers to treat patients without the supervision of a psychiatrist, however they were not allowed to collect payment for their services from insurance companies

22) This is a general term that refers to a type of severe mental disorder in which the individual is considered to be out of contact with reality.

    a. threshold

    b. syndrome

    c. psychosis

    d. schizophrenia

23) _____ is to experience as _____ is to genes.

    a. nature; nurture

    b. nurture; nature

    c. quantitative; qualitative

    d. qualitative; quantitative

24) The conclusion of Jane Murphy's study of the Inuit of northwest Alaska and the Yoruba of rural, tropical Nigeria was that:

   a. severe forms of mental illness are not limited to Western cultures or developed countries
   b. severe forms of mental illness do appear to be limited to Western cultures or developed countries
   c. severe forms of mental illness are more prevalent in Western cultures and developed countries
   d. severe forms of mental illness are more prevalent in the Inuit and Yoruba populations studied

25) In order for a behavior to be considered abnormal, it must include all of the following EXCEPT:

   a. present distress or painful symptoms
   b. conflicts between the individual and society that are voluntary in nature
   c. impairment in one or more important areas of functioning
   d. increased risk of suffering death, pain, disability, or an important loss of freedom

26) Which is true about the role of value judgments in the development of diagnostic systems?

   a. values can be avoided with the use of scientific methods
   b. diagnosis is completely determined by values
   c. values have no place in the attempt to define disease
   d. values are inherent in any attempt to define disease

27) Which of the following is a model that views psychopathology as resulting from physical factors that form a predisposition combined with a threatening or challenging experience?

   a. medical model
   b. diathesis-stress model
   c. threshold model
   d. biopsychosocial model

28) According to a national study conducted by the President's Commission on Mental Health, at least one in every _____ Americans exhibited active symptoms of at least one mental disorder during a specific 12-month period of time.

    a. 5
    b. 10
    c. 15
    d. 20

29) Olivia grew up in a society where mourners pull out their hair, go into an emotional frenzy, and begin speaking in tongues. On a visit to the U.S., she did these things in public when she heard that a relative had died. According to DSM-IV, this would be considered:

    a. not to be psychopathology, because it is part of her culture
    b. not to be psychopathology, because it caused no disruption in her social relationships
    c. to be psychopathology, because of her personal distress
    d. to be psychopathology, because it impaired her functioning

30) Which of the following is NOT considered a criterion for defining a behavior as a form of mental illness?

    a. negative effects on the person's social functioning
    b. recognition by the person that his or her behavior is problematic
    c. personal discomfort
    d. persistent, maladaptive behaviors

BRIEF ESSAY

As a final exercise, write out answers to the following brief essay questions. Then compare your answers with the material presented in the text.

After you have answered these questions, review the "Critical Thinking" questions that are presented at the end of the text chapter. Answering these questions will help you integrate important issues and themes that have been featured throughout the chapter.

1. Briefly describe the criteria that need to be present in order for a behavior to be considered "abnormal." Why is it important to have criteria in order to define a behavior as "abnormal?"

2. Compare and contrast the various approaches presented in this chapter that attempt to explain the etiology of abnormal behavior. What are the strengths and weaknesses of these models?

3. Choose one of the four case studies presented in this chapter and briefly describe the importance of the case in learning about the disorder. In what ways is this case similar to the other three cases? What are some issues that are unique to this case? What can be learned from studying case studies?

ANSWER KEY

MATCHING EXERCISES

1.	c	11.	f
2.	o	12.	p
3.	r	13.	g
4.	s	14.	b
5.	k	15.	l
6.	t	16.	e
7.	a	17.	m
8.	d	18.	h
9.	i	19.	n
10.	q	20.	j

MULTIPLE CHOICE EXERCISES

1.	a	20.	b
2.	d	21.	a
3.	c	22.	c
4.	c	23.	b
5.	b	24.	a
6.	a	25.	b
7.	b	26.	d
8.	d	27.	b
9.	c	28.	a
10.	b	29.	a
11.	b	30.	b
12.	a		
13.	d		
14.	a		
15.	b		
16.	d		
17.	c		
18.	a		
19.	d		

CHAPTER TWO
CAUSES OF ABNORMAL BEHAVIOR: FROM PARADIGMS TO SYSTEMS

CHAPTER OUTLINE

Overview
    Brief Historical Perspective
        General Paresis and the Biological Approach
        Freud and the Psychoanalytic Approach
        Free Will and the Humanistic Approach
    Paradigms and the Causes of Abnormal Behavior

Systems Theory
    Holism
        Reductionism
    Subsystems and Levels of Analysis
        Abnormalities and Causality across Subsystems
    Common Processes within Different Levels of Analysis
    Development

Biological Factors
    The Neuron
        Neurotransmitters and the Etiology of Psychopathology
    Major Brain Structures
        Psychophysiology and the Etiology of Psychopathology
        Major Brain Structures and the Etiology of Psychopathology
    Psychophysiology
        Endocrine System
        Nervous System
    Behavior Genetics
        Some Basic Principles of Genetics
        Adoption Studies
        Family Incidence Studies
        Misinterpreting Behavior Genetics Findings
        Twin Studies
        Genetics and the Etiology of Psychopathology

Psychological Factors
    Basic Motivations and Temperamental Styles
        Hierarchy of Needs
        Attachment Theory
        Dominance Relations
        Emotions and Emotional Systems

Temperament
Basic Motivation, Temperament, and the Etiology of
Psychopathology
Learning and Cognition
Modeling
Social Cognition
Learning, Distorted Cognition, and the Etiology of
Psychopathology
The Sense of Self
Self Systems and the Etiology of Psychopathology

Stages of Development
Development and the Etiology of Psychopathology

Social Factors
Relationships and Psychopathology
Marital Status and Psychopathology
Social Relationships
Gender and Gender Roles
Race and Poverty
"Sick" Societies

Summary

LEARNING OBJECTIVES

After reviewing the material presented in this chapter, you should be able to:

*   define the biopsychosocial approach and explain how it is a systems approach

*   name some of the major breakthroughs that led to modern scientific abnormal
psychology:
a) discovery of the biological origins of general paresis,
b) Freud's talking cure with hysterical patients, and
c) emergence of scientific academic psychology (Wundt, Pavlov, Skinner, Watson,
etc.)

*   distinguish holism from reductionism

*   describe the basic functions of the hindbrain, midbrain, and forebrain

*   separate central from peripheral nervous systems; voluntary vs. autonomic nervous
systems; sympathetic vs. parasympathetic nervous system

14

*   know the basic research design used for twin studies, adoption studies, and family incidence studies

*   define temperament and explain its significance in the etiology of psychopathology

*   describe some ways in which modeling, social cognition, and sense of self may affect abnormal behavior

*   understand that the following social factors are generally correlated (not causative) with psychopathology: relationship difficulties, gender, race, and poverty

KEY TERMS AND CONCEPTS

Following is a list of key terms and concepts that are featured in the chapter and are important for you to know. Write out the definitions of each of these terms and check your answers with the definitions in the text.

Etiology
Paradigm
Multifactorial causes
Nature-nurture debate
Biopsychosocial
Biological Approach
General paresis
Syphilis
Arsphenamine
Psychoanalytic Approach
Hysteria
The unconscious
Id
Libido
Pleasure principle
Ego
Reality principle
Superego
Neurotic anxiety
Defense mechanisms
Theory of psychosexual development
Oedipal conflict
Electra complex
Introspection
Classical conditioning

Unconditioned stimulus
Unconditioned response
Conditioned stimulus
Conditioned response
Extinction
Operant conditioning
Positive reinforcement
Negative reinforcement
Punishment
Response cost
Contingency
Behaviorism
Denial
Displacement
Projection
Rationalization
Reaction formation
Repression
Sublimation
Humanistic psychology
Free will
Medical model
Systems theory
Holism
Reductionism
Subsystems
Molecular
Molar
Levels of analysis
Reciprocal causality
Linear causality
Cybernetics
Hemostasis
Developmental psychopathology
Developmental norms
Premorbid history
Prognosis
Anatomy
Physiology
Neuroanatomy
Neurophysiology
Neurons
Soma
Dendrites

Axon
Terminal Buttons
Synapse
Receptors
Reuptake
Neuromodulators
Endorphins
Opoids
Dualism
Hindbrain
Medulla
Pons
Cerebellum
Midbrain
Reticular activating system
Forebrain
Limbic system
Thalamus
Hypothalamus
Cerebral hemispheres
Lateralized
Corpus callosum
Ventricles
Cerebral cortex
Psychophysiology
Endocrine system
Hormones
Hyperthyroidism/Graves' disease
Central nervous system
Peripheral nervous system
Somatic nervous system
Autonomic nervous system
Sympathetic nervous system
Parasympathetic nervous system
Genes
Chromosomes
Behavior genetics
Genotype
Phenotype
Alleles
Locus
Polygenic
Monozygotic (MZ)
Dizygotic (DZ)

Probands
Predestination
Individual differences
Species-typical characteristics
Hierarchy of needs
Self-actualization
Attachment Theory
Imprinting
Dominance
Temperament
Temperamental styles
The Big Five
Extraversion
Agreeableness
Conscientiousness
Neuroticism
Openness to experience
Anxious attachments
Goodness of fit
Modeling
Identification
Social cognition
Attributions
Learned helplessness theory
Cognitive errors
Identity
Role identities
Self-schema
Irrational beliefs
Self-control
Socialization
Self-concept
Self-efficacy
Stage of development
Developmental transition
Fixation
Regression
Social roles
Labeling theory
Self-fulfilling prophesy
Correlational study

Social support
Gender roles
Androgyny
Cultural relativity

KEY NAMES

The following individuals have made important contributions to the material presented in the chapter. Write out the names of these individuals and the theories, research, or treatment with which they are associated. Then check your answers with the information in your text.

Hippocrates
Sigmund Freud
Jean Charcot
Wilhelm Wundt
Ivan Pavlov
B.F. Skinner
John B. Watson
Abraham Maslow
Frederich (Fritz) Perls
Carl Rogers
Thomas Kuhn
Ludwig von Bertalanffy
Rene' Descartes
Gregor Mendel
John Bowlby
Harry Stack Sullivan
Erik Erikson
Albert Bandura
George Kelly
Albert Ellis
Jean Piaget

MATCHING QUESTIONS

Match the following terms and names with the definitions presented below. The answers can be found at the end of the chapter.

a. molecular
b. autonomic nervous system
c. displacement
d. soma

k. repression
l. Ivan Pavlov
m. peripheral nervous system
n. reductionism

19

e. dualism
f. Wilhelm Wundt
g. central nervous system
h. psychoanalytic approach
i. endocrine system
j. John B. Watson

o. biological approach
p. terminal button
q. molar
r. paradigm
s. sanguine (cheerful)
t. Ludwig von Bertalanffy

1) _____ he founded behaviorism, arguing that observable behavior was the only appropriate subject matter for the science of psychology

2) _____ includes the substance of a theory as well as a set of assumptions about how scientists should collect data and test theoretical propositions

3) _____ this approach can be traced back to the study of general paresis

4) _____ the most general explanation

5) _____ the defense mechanism where feelings or actions are transferred from one person or object to another that is less threatening

6) _____ according to Hippocrates, this type of personality was caused by an excess of blood

7) _____ the cell body and largest part of the neuron

8) _____ the idea that the task for scientists is to divide the world into its smaller and smaller components

9) _____ in his famous experiments on classical conditioning, he rang a bell every time he fed meat powder to dogs

10) _____ his goal was to understand consciousness through a technique called introspection

11) _____ a collection of glands found at various locations throughout the body

12) _____ a bud found on the small branches at the end of the axon where messages are sent to other neurons

13) _____ includes all connections that stem out from the brain and spinal cord and innervate the body's muscles, sensory system, and organs

14) ____ is divided into the sympathetic nervous system and the parasympathetic nervous system

15) ____ includes the brain and spinal cord

16) ____ considered to be the "father of systems theory"

17) ____ the philosophical view that the mind and body are somehow separable

18) ____ the most reductionistic explanation

19) ____ owes its origins to the writings of Sigmund Freud

20) ____ the defense mechanism in which threatening material is suppressed from consciousness, although you don't deny the memory when reminded of it

MULTIPLE CHOICE QUESTIONS

The following multiple choice questions will test your comprehension of the material presented in the chapter. Circle the correct choice for each question in the section. Then compare your answers with those at the end of the chapter.

1) This nervous system regulates the functions of various body organs such as the heart and stomach.

    a. somatic nervous system
    b. autonomic nervous system
    c. sympathetic nervous system
    d. parasympathetic nervous system

2) According to Freud, this is the part of the personality that attempts to fulfill id impulses while at the same time dealing with the realities of the world.

    a. ego
    b. id
    c. superego
    d. libido

3) All of the following are methods of learning EXCEPT:

    a. classical conditioning
    b. operant conditioning
    c. introjection

d. modeling

4) Leading developmental theory speculates that children whose parents are _____ and _____ are better adjusted than those whose parents are inadequate on one or both of these dimensions.

    a. loving; firm in their discipline
    b. authoritative; hold high expectations of their child
    c. demanding; promote individuality
    d. congenial; encourage separation and independence

5) Freud was trained by this neurologist who successfully used hypnosis to treat what used to be called hysteria.

    a. Harry Stack Sullivan
    b. Ludwig von Bertalanffy
    c. Fritz Perls
    d. Jean Charcot

6) While watching her daughter play kickball in the street of their neighborhood, Mrs. Jones witnesses her daughter fatally being hit by a car. Shortly following this tragedy, Mrs. Jones loses her vision. After visits to numerous doctors, there is no known organic impairment to cause the blindness. Mrs. Jones' condition could be considered which of the following disorders?

    a. depression
    b. conversion disorder
    c. hysteria
    d. hypochondriasis

7) Which of the following could be considered an uncertain or ambivalent parent-child relationship that is a consequence of inconsistent and unresponsive parenting, particularly during the first year of life?

    a. anxious attachment
    b. neurotic attachment
    c. oppositional attachment
    d. apathetic attachment

8) All of the following are associated with the humanistic approach EXCEPT:

    a. Carl Rogers
    b. B.F. Skinner
    c. Fritz Perls

d. Abraham Maslow

9) In the famous experiments on which classical conditioning was based, the bell served as the _____ and the meat powder was the _____.

 a. conditioned response; unconditioned response
 b. unconditioned response; conditioned response
 c. conditioned stimulus; unconditioned stimulus
 d. unconditioned stimulus; conditioned stimulus

10) The enigma written by Lord Byron and presented in this chapter illustrates that:

 a. paradigms are unscientific and therefore should not be used in evaluating situations
 b. the hidden meanings in life are sometimes difficult to comprehend, however the use of a paradigm can aid in this process
 c. we should use our paradigm to help reveal the meaning from certain situations
 d. assumptions made by a paradigm can at times act as blinders and lead an investigator to overlook what otherwise might be obvious

11) Mike's mother took away his privilege to use the computer for two days because he hit his sister. This is an example of:

 a. punishment
 b. response cost
 c. extinction
 d. negative reinforcement

12) Systems theory has roots in all of the following EXCEPT:

 a. biology
 b. engineering
 c. philosophy
 d. all of the above

13) _____ are chainlike structures that are found in the nucleus of cells.

 a. alleles
 b. genes
 c. chromosomes
 d. loci

14) Which of the following is a pattern of behavior that precedes the onset of the disorder?

a. prognosis
b. premorbid history
c. determinism
d. self-fulfilling prophesy

15) Advances in the scientific understanding of the etiology of psychopathology did not appear until the nineteenth and early twentieth centuries when all of the following major events occurred EXCEPT:

a. the number of people diagnosed with some form of psychopathology rapidly increased
b. the cause of general paresis was discovered
c. the emergence of Sigmund Freud
d. the creation of a new academic discipline called psychology

16) According to Freud's theory of psychosexual development, boys harboring forbidden sexual desires for their mothers is called (a/an):

a. defense mechanism
b. neurotic anxiety
c. Electra complex
d. Oedipal conflict

17) According to the "Big Five" bipolar dimensions of personality, this domain is characterized by trusting and kind versus hostile and selfish.

a. conscientiousness
b. agreeableness
c. neuroticism
d. extraversion

18) According to the psychodynamic paradigm, the cause of abnormality is:

a. early childhood experiences
b. social learning
c. frustrations of society
d. genes, infection, or other physical damage

19) The cornerstone of humanistic psychology, _____ is the assumption that human behavior is not determined but is a product of how people choose to act.

a. holism
b. self-fulfilling prophesy

c. individuation

d. free will

20) Which of the following is a communication and control process that uses feedback loops to adjust progress toward a goal?

a. homeostasis

b. neuromodulators

c. cybernetics

d. neurotransmitters

21) This nervous system is responsible for controlling activities associated with increased arousal and energy expenditure.

a. sympathetic nervous system

b. parasympathetic nervous system

c. autonomic nervous system

d. somatic nervous system

22) Which of the following terms represents a conclusion that a psychological disorder will inevitably appear if it has a genetic component?

a. self-fulfilling prophesy

b. self-actualization

c. predestination

d. mediating process

23) Freud can be credited with all of the following EXCEPT:

a. offering specific, empirically-derived hypotheses about his theory

b. calling attention to unconscious processes

c. formulating a stage theory of child development

d. identifying numerous intrapsychic defenses

24) Which of the following are characteristic ways of behaving according to the expectations of the social situation?

a. prescribed roles

b. social roles

c. gender roles

d. transitional roles

25) All of the following are true from a systems perspective regarding the etiology of psychopathology EXCEPT:

    a. there may be biopsychosocial contributions to psychopathology, but clear hypotheses must still be supported by empirical evidence
    b. social domains of behavior are the most significant contribution to the causes of abnormal behavior
    c. different types of abnormal behavior have very different causes
    d. causes of almost all forms of abnormal behavior are unknown at present

26) According to the behavioral paradigm, the inborn human nature is:

    a. aggressive
    b. basically good
    c. basically selfish, but having some altruism
    d. neutral, like a blank slate

27) Which of the following is a defense mechanism that includes the insistence that an experience, memory, or internal need did not occur or does not exist?

    a. sublimation
    b. reaction formation
    c. denial
    d. repression

28) This occurs when a conditioned stimulus is no longer presented together with an unconditioned stimulus.

    a. extinction
    b. punishment
    c. negative reinforcement
    d. response cost

29) A _____ is an individual's actual genetic structure.

    a. locus
    b. phenotype
    c. proband
    d. genotype

30) This theory suggests that depression is caused by wrongly attributing bad events to internal, global, and stable causes.

    a. labeling theory

b. learned helplessness theory
c. modeling theory
d. social cognition theory

BRIEF ESSAY

As a final exercise, write out answers to the following brief essay questions. Then compare your answers with the material presented in the text.

After you have answered these questions, review the "Critical Thinking" questions that are presented at the end of the text chapter. Answering these questions will help you integrate important issues and themes that have been featured throughout the chapter.

1. Compare and contrast the following behavior genetics investigations: twin studies, adoption, and family incidence studies. In what ways are these findings helpful? In what ways could these findings possibly be misinterpreted?

2. Discuss Maslow's hierarchy of needs theory. In what ways is this similar to attachment theory as proposed by Bowlby? In what ways is it different? Could these theories complement one another? Why or why not?

3. Compare and contrast Freud and Erikson's theories on development. Which theory makes the most sense to you and your personal experience? Why?

4. Discuss why it is not enough to focus on one subsystem or level of analysis when viewing psychopathology. What do you gain by focusing on multifactorial causes?

ANSWER KEY

MATCHING EXERCISES

1. j	11. i
2. r	12. p
3. o	13. m
4. q	14. b
5. c	15. g
6. s	16. t
7. d	17. e
8. n	18. a
9. l	19. h
10. f	20. k

MULTIPLE CHOICE EXERCISES

1. b	6. b	11. b
2. a	7. a	12. d
3. c	8. b	13. c
4. a	9. c	14. b
5. d	10. d	15. a

16. d	21. a	26. d
17. b	22. c	27. c
18. a	23. a	28. a
19. d	24. b	29. d
20. c	25. b	30. b

CHAPTER THREE
TREATMENT OF PSYCHOLOGICAL DISORDERS

CHAPTER OUTLINE

Overview

Pragmatic Approaches to Psychotherapy
    Brief Historical Perspective
    Biological Treatments
        Electroconvulsive Therapy (ECT)
        Psychosurgery
        Psychopharmacology
    Psychodynamic Psychotherapies
        Freudian Psychoanalysis
            Current Status of Freudian Psychoanalysis
        Ego Analysis
            Attachment Theory
        Psychodynamic Psychotherapy
            Short-Term Psychodynamic Psychotherapy
    Behavior Therapy
        Classical Conditioning Techniques
            Systematic Desensitization
            In Vivo Desensitization
            Flooding
            Aversion Therapy
        Operant Conditioning Techniques
            Contingency Management
            Social Skills Training
    Cognitive-Behavior Therapy
        Attribution Therapy
        Self-Instruction Training
        Cognitive Therapy
        Rational-Emotive Therapy (RET)
    Humanistic Therapies
        Client-Centered Therapy
        Gestalt Therapy
        Existential Analysis

Research on Psychotherapy
    Psychotherapy Outcome Research
        Meta-Analysis
        Improvement without Treatment
        Outcome Research on Different Schools of Psychotherapy

Psychotherapy Process Research
The Placebo Effect
Psychotherapy as Social Support
Psychotherapy as Social Influence

Changing Social Systems: Couples, Family, and Group Therapy
Couples Therapy
Family Therapy
Group Therapy
Community Psychology and Prevention

Developing Specific Treatments for Specific Disorders

Summary

LEARNING OBJECTIVES

After reviewing the material presented in this chapter, you should be able to:

*   make broad comparisons between biological, psychodynamic, behavioral, and humanistic approaches to treatment

*   distinguish the two historical trends towards spiritual/religious treatment from the natural/scientific approach to treatment

*   describe electroconvulsive therapy and psychosurgery as they are practiced today

*   evaluate the overall effectiveness of psychopharmacology in the treatment of mental illness

*   describe the basic goals and primary techniques involved in psychoanalysis

*   explain the theory behind ego analysis and the differences between psychoanalysis and psychodynamic psychotherapy

*   articulate the ways in which classical conditioning principles are utilized in such behavior therapy techniques as systematic desensitization, in vivo desensitization, flooding, and aversion therapy

*   describe contingency management and social skills training programs

*   understand the basic principles of attribution therapy, self-instruction training, cognitive therapy, and rational emotive therapy

*   know how each of the humanistic therapies--client-centered therapy, gestalt therapy, and existential analysis--reflects the underlying principles of humanistic psychology

*   describe the basic findings produced from meta-analysis of psychotherapy outcome studies

*   use Sloane's study to compare behavioral therapy with psychodynamic psychotherapy in terms of outcomes

*   define psychotherapy process research and describe some of its basic findings

*   compare the goals, techniques, and known outcomes of couples therapy, family therapy, and group therapy; describe the differences between these approaches and individual psychotherapy

*   list some basic recommendations that the authors suggest will improve the effectiveness of psychotherapy

KEY TERMS AND CONCEPTS

Following is a list of key terms and concepts that are featured in the chapter and are important for you to know. Write out the definitions of each of these terms and check your answers with the definitions in the text.

Psychotherapy
Psychotherapy outcome research
Psychotherapy process research
Eclectic
Biological therapies
Psychodynamic therapies
Behavior therapies
Cognitive therapies
Humanistic therapies
Defensive style
Homework
Genuineness
Trephining
Experiment
Hypothesis
Independent variable
Random assignment
Dependent variable
Statistically significant
Internal validity

External validity
Symptom alleviation
Electroconvulsive therapy (ECT)
Bilateral ECT
Unilateral ECT
Psychosurgery
Prefrontal lobotomy
Placebo control group
Informed consent
Psychopharmacology
Psychoactive drugs
Cathartic method or Catharsis
Free association
Psychoanalysis
Insight
Interpretation
Therapeutic neutrality
Transference
Countertransference
Psychodynamic
Ego analysis
Short-term psychodynamic psychotherapy
Behaviorism
Counterconditioning
Progressive muscle relaxation
Hierarchy of fears
In vivo desensitization
Flooding
Aversion therapy
Rapid smoking technique
Contingency management
Token economy
Social skills training
Assertiveness training
Social problem solving
Cognitive-behavior therapy
Attribution therapy
Self-instruction therapy
Collaborative empiricism
Rational-emotive therapy (RET)
Emotional awareness
Client-centered therapy
Empathy
Self-disclosure

Unconditional positive regard
Gestalt therapy
Empty chair technique
Existential analysis
Process research
Meta-analysis
Spontaneous remission
Placebo effect
Dissonance
Couples therapy
Communication
Negotiation skills/conflict resolution
Family therapy
Parent management training
Alliances
Group therapy
Psychoeducational groups
Experiential group therapy
Self-help groups
Paraprofessionals
Community psychology
Primary prevention
Secondary prevention
Tertiary prevention
Applied relaxation
Nondirective therapy

KEY NAMES

The following individuals have made important contributions to the material presented in the chapter. Write out the names of these individuals and the theories, research, or treatment with which they are associated. Then check your answers with the information in your text.

Hippocrates
Ugo Cerletti
Lucio Bini
Egas Moniz
Joseph Breuer
Sigmund Freud
Harry Stack Sullivan
Erik Erikson
Karen Horney

John Bowlby
John B. Watson
Joseph Wolpe
Ivan Pavlov
B.F. Skinner
Albert Bandura
Aaron Beck
Albert Ellis
Carl Rogers
Frederich (Fritz) Perls
Ludwig Binswanger
Medard Boss
Rollo May
Hans Eysenck
Jerome Frank
Thomas Bokovac
Ellen Costello

MATCHING QUESTIONS

Match the following terms and names with the definitions presented below. The answers can be found at the end of the chapter.

a. independent variable
b. experiential group therapy
c. cognitive therapy
d. psychoeducational group
e. primary prevention
f. psychotherapy outcome research
g. biological therapy
h. self-help group
i. gestalt therapy
j. psychotherapy process research

k. Erik Erikson
l. behavior therapy
m. psychodynamic therapy
n. insight
o. John Bowlby
p. dependent variable
q. secondary prevention
r. interpretation
s. countertransference
t. transference

1) _____ analyst brings formerly unconscious material into conscious awareness

2) _____ helps clients to recognize and accept their emotional experiences by encouraging them to live in the "here and now"

3) _____ the variable that is hypothesized to vary or to change

4) _____ group that focuses on the relationships between group members

34

5) _____ process whereby patients project their feelings about some key figure in their life onto the analyst

6) _____ improvement of the environment in order to prevent new cases of a mental disorder from developing

7) _____ his interest in studying close relationships early in life greatly contributed to attachment theory

8) _____ emphasizes the application of basic psychological research to the treatment of psychological disorders

9) _____ the early detection of emotional problems in the hope of preventing them from becoming more serious and difficult to treat

10) _____ typically not considered a therapy group, this type of group brings people together who share a common problem

11) _____ the variable that is deliberately controlled and manipulated by the experimenter

12) _____ developed specifically for depression, the goal of this type of therapy is to challenge the clients' negative distortions of the world and of themselves

13) _____ his theory of development emphasized psychosocial stages of development

14) _____ process whereby the analyst lets his or her own feelings influence his or her responses to a patient

15) _____ compares the effectiveness of alternative forms of treatment

16) _____ analysts suggests hidden meanings to patients' accounts of their past and present life

17) _____ treatment approach that understands mental illness by drawing an analogy to physical illness

18) _____ group designed to teach members specific information or skills relevant to psychological well-being

19) _____ treatment that typically begins with an exploration of the client's past, unconscious motivations, and defense mechanisms

20) _____ investigates similarities in practice by studying aspects of the client-therapist relationship

MULTIPLE CHOICE QUESTIONS

The following multiple choice questions will test your comprehension of the material presented in the chapter. Circle the correct choice for each question in the section. Then compare your answers with those at the end of the chapter.

1) According to attribution theory, depressed people often attribute _____ to themselves and _____ to others.

    a. success; failure
    b. failure; success
    c. irrational beliefs; rational beliefs
    d. rational beliefs; irrational beliefs

2) Treatment outcome researchers widely accept the finding that approximately _____ of clients improve as a result of psychotherapy.

    a. one-third
    b. two-thirds
    c. one-quarter
    d. one-half

3) Empathy involves:

    a. trying to put yourself in someone else's shoes in order to understand their feelings and perspectives
    b. trying to understand the etiology of someone else's behavior
    c. feeling sorry for someone because of their life situation
    d. all of the above

4) The "placebo effect" is:

    a. treatment in which the client has a dialogue with an imagined part of himself or herself
    b. treatment in which the client is taught relaxation skills for the condition being evaluated
    c. treatment that contains no "special ingredient" for treating the condition being evaluated
    d. treatment which involves full intensity exposure to feared stimuli

5) Every day that Sally completes all of her chores at home her mother gives her a star. After Sally has accumulated 15 stars, her mother will take her out for ice cream. Sally's mother is most likely using which of the following to get Sally to do her chores?

     a. token economy
     b. counterconditioning
     c. in vivo desensitization
     d. classical conditioning

6) The core theme of the existential analysis approach to treatment is:

     a. helping the client to identify problem areas in his or her life and
        work toward changing these
     b. helping the client to find meaning in life
     c. helping the client to learn to express his or her unconscious drives
        and conflicts
     d. helping the client to be genuine and self-accepting

7) Which of the following would most likely ask a patient to do homework?

     a. a biological therapist
     b. a psychodynamic therapist
     c. a humanistic therapist
     d. a behavior therapist

8) Electroconvulsive therapy (ECT) was originally used based on the erroneous assumption that
     a. resulting memory loss would cure schizophrenia.
     b. schizophrenia was located in one hemisphere of the brain.
     c. schizophrenia prevented epileptic seizures.
     d. epileptic seizures prevented schizophrenia.

9) All of the following are examples of behavior therapy EXCEPT:

     a. flooding
     b. social skills training
     c. aversion therapy
     d. empty chair technique

10) An experiment has internal validity if:

     a. the findings can be generalized to other circumstances
     b. changes in the dependent variable can be accurately attributed to
        changes in the independent variable

    c. the researcher can control virtually every aspect of the experimental
      environment
    d. the researcher is able to control and manipulate the dependent
      variable

11) This type of therapy is primarily used to treat substance abuse disorders such as alcoholism and cigarette smoking.

    a. cognitive therapy
    b. psychodynamic therapy
    c. aversion therapy
    d. contingency therapy

12) Sam is a first-year college student who is extremely afraid of heights. He entered therapy after failing his first semester chemistry course because it was located on the fifth floor of a building, and Sam was too afraid to go the fifth floor to attend class. Sam's therapist gradually exposes Sam to increasing heights in a natural setting while having Sam simultaneously maintain a state of relaxation. Sam's therapist is using which technique to help Sam alleviate his fear of heights?

    a. in vivo desensitization
    b. systematic desensitization
    c. flooding
    d. countercondioning

13) Albert Ellis is to _____ as Aaron Beck is to _____.

    a. client-centered therapy; ego analysis
    b. ego analysis; client-centered therapy
    c. rational-emotive therapy; cognitive therapy
    d. cognitive therapy; rational-emotive therapy

14) According to Sigmund Freud, all of the following are ways to reveal aspects of the unconscious mind EXCEPT:

    a. slips of the tongue
    b. countertransference
    c. dreams
    d. free association

15) One major difference in technique between humanistic and behavior therapists is:

    a. humanistic psychotherapists view the nature of the therapist-client
      relationship differently than behavior therapists

b. humanistic psychotherapists focus on the patients' past and present interpersonal relationships

c. humanistic psychotherapists focus on treatment irrespective of its causes

d. all of the above

16) All of the following have caused a decline in the practice of classical Freudian psychoanalysis EXCEPT:

a. the substantial amount of time required

b. the accessibility of treatment only by those who are relatively financially secure

c. research has proven classical Freudian psychoanalysis to be ineffective

d. the limited data available on the outcome of treatment

17) In the 1990s this medication has outsold every prescription medication, including all medications used to treat physical ailments.

a. Valium

b. Prozac

c. Ritalin

d. Lithium

18) All of the following can be viewed as goals of psychoanalysis EXCEPT:

a. to rid the patient of his or her defenses

b. to increase self-understanding

c. to bring unconscious material into conscious awareness

d. to release pent-up emotions and unexpressed feelings

19) Pavlov is to _____ as Skinner is to _____.

a. in vivo desensitization; systematic desensitization

b. systematic desensitization; in vivo desensitization

c. operant conditioning; classical conditioning

d. classical conditioning; operant conditioning

20) Psychotherapy outcome research indicates that:

a. clients who are young, attractive, verbal, intelligent, and successful tend to improve more in psychotherapy

b. if psychotherapy is going to be effective, it will be effective rather quickly

c. psychotherapy is generally effective when compared with no treatment
   at all
d. all of the above

21) Collaborative empiricism involves:

   a. relieving a clients' symptoms through the use of medication
   b. revealing aspects of a clients' unconscious drives and conflicts
   c. confronting a clients' unrealistic feelings about himself/herself
   d. challenging a clients' negative distortions

22) Aversion therapy is a type of:

   a. classical conditioning technique
   b. operant conditioning technique
   c. cognitive-behavioral technique
   d. social skills training technique

23) An ancient practice called trephining sought to treat mental illness by:

   a. dunking suspected witches in the water
   b. confining patients in insane asylums
   c. chipping a hole in the skull to let spirits escape
   d. performing sacrifices

24) Research indicates that _____ is the most effective approach to treating
psychological disorders.

   a. humanistic psychotherapy
   b. psychodynamic psychotherapy
   c. existential psychotherapy
   d. research generally reveals few differences among approaches

25) The term "unconditional positive regard" refers to:

   a. valuing a client for who they are and refraining from judging them
   b. only making positive comments to a client and never devaluing them as
      a human being
   c. the relationship between the client and therapist
   d. none of the above

26) _____ has been the most promising avenue of biological treatment.

   a. psychosurgery

b. classical conditioning
c. operant conditioning
d. psychopharmacology

27) In order for a finding to be statistically significant at the .05 level of significance, it would need to occur by chance alone in:

a. 1 out of every 5 experiments
b. 1 out of every 10 experiments
c. 1 out of every 15 experiments
d. 1 out of every 20 experiments

28) All of the following were primary contributors to the field of humanistic therapies EXCEPT:

a. Carl Rogers
b. Albert Bandura
c. Fritz Perls
d. Rollo May

29) _____ is used in training clients to use relaxation techniques to cope with thoughts, feelings, or situations that provoke anxiety.

a. secondary relaxation
b. emotional relaxation
c. applied relaxation
d. primary relaxation

30) This method became the cornerstone of Freud's psychoanalysis.

a. free association
b. hypnosis
c. catharsis
d. interpretation

BRIEF ESSAY

As a final exercise, write out answers to the following brief essay questions. Then compare your answers with the material presented in the text.

After you have answered these questions, review the "Critical Thinking" questions that are presented at the end of the text chapter. Answering these questions will help you integrate important issues and themes that have been featured throughout the chapter.

1. Compare and contrast the biological, psychodynamic, behavioral, and humanistic approaches to treating psychological disorders. In what ways might these approaches be similar in working with a patient diagnosed with depression? In what ways might they be different?

2. Discuss how the ideas of ego analysts differ from the original ideas of Freud. In what ways are they still similar?

3. Discuss some of the ethical concerns that psychologists have encountered in the past. What are some ways in which ethical issues are now being handled in the field of psychology?

ANSWER KEY

MATCHING EXERCISES

1. n	11. a
2. i	12. c
3. p	13. k
4. b	14. s
5. t	15. f
6. e	16. r
7. o	17. g
8. l	18. d
9. q	19. m
10. h	20. j

MULTIPLE CHOICE EXERCISES

1. b	6. b	11. c
2. b	7. d	12. a
3. a	8. d	13. c
4. c	9. d	14. b
5. a	10. b	15. a

16. c	21. d	26. d
17. b	22. a	27. d
18. a	23. c	28. b
19. d	24. d	29. c
20. d	25. a	30. a

CHAPTER FOUR
CLASSIFICATION AND ASSESSMENT

CHAPTER OUTLINE

Overview
      Issues and Choices

Basic Issues in Classification
      Categories Versus Dimensions
      Monothetic Versus Polythetic Classes
      Description Versus Theory

Classification of Abnormal Behavior
      Brief Historical Perspective
      The DSM-IV System
            Diagnostic Axes

Evaluation of Classification Systems
      Reliability
      Validity
            The Relationship Between Reliability and Validity
      Unresolved Questions
      Nonscientific Factors that Affect Diagnostic Systems
            Professional Issues
      Laypeople and Political Organizations

Basic Issues in Assessment
      The Purposes of Clinical Assessment
      Assumptions About Behavior
            Consistency of Behavior
            Levels of Analysis
      Evaluation the Utility of Assessment Procedures

Assessment Procedures
      Assessment of Psychological Systems
            Interviews
                  Structured Interviews
                  Advantages
                  Limitations
            Observational Procedures
                  Rating Scales
                  Behavioral Coding Systems
                  Advantages

LEARNING OBJECTIVES

After reviewing the material presented in this chapter, you should be able to:

* define classification system, assessment, and diagnosis

* distinguish between a categorical approach to classification and a dimensional approach

* compare monothetic and polythetic classes

* explain why DSM-III represented a turning point in the diagnosis of psychiatric disorders

* describe the five axes used in diagnosis in DSM-IV

* understand the meaning and implications of reliability and validity in diagnosis and classification

* identify some of the advantages and also limitations of interview data for purposes of assessment

*   compare the three types of observational procedures--informal observations, rating scales, and behavioral coding systems

*   describe the strengths and weaknesses of the MMPI

*   list some of the advantages as well as limitations of using projective tests for assessment and diagnosis

*   identify the two methods employed for the assessment of social systems

*   describe two uses of psychophysiological assessment procedures and two limitations of this approach

*   compare static brain imaging techniques with dynamic brain imaging techniques in terms of the type of data each provides

KEY TERMS AND CONCEPTS

Following is a list of key terms and concepts that are featured in the chapter and are important for you to know. Write out the definitions of each of these terms and check your answers with the definitions in the text.

Asssessment
Classification system
Diagnosis
Dimensional approach to classification
Monothetic class
Polythetic class
Phenylketonuria (PKU)
Dementia praecox
Manic-depressive psychosis
International Classification of Diseases (ICD)
Diagnostic and Statistical Manual of Mental Disorders (DSM)
Labeling theory
Multiaxial
Inclusion criteria
Exclusion criteria
Reliability
Kappa coefficient
Validity
Etiological validity
Concurrent validity
Predictive validity

Self-defeating personality disorder
Test-retest reliability
Split-half reliability
False positives
Sensitivity
Specificity
Positive predictive power
Diagnostic efficiency
Structured interviews
Informal observations
Behavioral coding systems
Self-monitoring
Reactivity
Standardized
Validity scales
Actuarial
Unconscious
Somatic nervous system
Autonomic nervous system
Penile plethysmograph
Vaginal plethysmograph
Person variables
Situational variables
Computerized tomographic (CT) scanning
Magnetic resonance imaging (MRI)
Regional cerebral blood flow (rCBF)
Photons
Positron emission tomography (PET)

KEY NAMES

The following individuals have made important contributions to the material presented in the chapter. Write out the names of these individuals and the theories, research, or treatment with which they are associated. Then check your answers with the information in your text.

Carolus Linnaeus
Emil Kraeplin
Thomas Scheff
Robert Spitzer
Hermann Rorschach
John Exner

MATCHING QUESTIONS

Match the following terms and names with the definitions presented below. The answers can be found at the end of the chapter.

a. concurrent validity
b. reactivity
c. test-retest reliability
d. monothetic class
e. plethysmograph
f. structured interview
g. Hermann Rorschach
h. self-monitoring
i. sensitivity
j. exclusion criteria

k. diagnostic efficiency
l. Robert Spitzer
m. specificity
n. predictive validity
o. polythetic class
p. electrocardiogram
q. inter-rater reliability
r. kappa
s. assessment
t. phenulketonuria (PKU)

1) _____ the general process of information gathering, which can include the use of a variety of specific tools and procedures

2) _____ a Swiss psychiatrist who developed a well-known projective test

3) _____ a method of assessing the consistency of decisions across interviewers or raters

4) _____ defining a category using a number of characteristics that are considered singly necessary and jointly sufficient

5) _____ concerned with the ability of a measure to accurately assess the presence of a disorder that would manifest itself at some time in the future

6) _____ an inherited metabolic disorder that can produce mental retardation

7) _____ concerned with the ability of a test to accurately identify individuals who have the particular disorder in question

8) _____ a prominent psychiatrist conducting research in psychiatric classification and who chaired the committee responsible for developing the DSM-III

9) _____ a method of assessing the consistency of a measure over time

10) _____ a procedure in which the clinician must ask each person a specific

list of detailed questions, usually in a specific order, in order to gather diagnostic information

11) _____ each member of this type of category must possess a specified minimal number of the defining characteristics

12) _____ an instrument that assesses the engorgement of genital tissue with blood

13) _____ a statistical measure used to assess reliability of psychiatric diagnosis

14) _____ criteria included in a diagnostic category that are concerned with ruling out the presence of other diagnoses

15) _____ concerned with the ability of a test to accurately identify the individuals who do NOT have the particular disorder in question

16) _____ a procedure used by adults that allows them to keep track of one or more of their behaviors that they are systematically observing

17) _____ concerned with the ability of a measure to accurately assess the presence of a disorder at the present time

18) _____ refers to the overall ability of a test to make correct and incorrect predictions about individuals

19) _____ a type of procedure that assesses the action potential of cardiac muscle during contraction

20) _____ changes that occur in a person's behavior because of the process of being observed

MULTIPLE CHOICE QUESTIONS

The following multiple choice questions will test your comprehension of the material presented in the chapter. Circle the correct choice for each question in the section. Then compare your answers with those at the end of the chapter.

1) A definitive characteristic of ALL projective tests is:

    a. a true-false response format
    b. the use of a list of open-ended sentences that the individual must answer

c. the use of items describing various thoughts, feelings, and behaviors
   that the individual must rate
d. the use of ambiguous stimuli

2) Which approach to classification is based on an ordered sequence or on quantative measurements rather than qualitative judgments?

   a. dimensional approach
   b. categorical approach
   c. diagnostic approach
   d. monothetic approach

3) Which of the following is NOT an axis of DSM-IV?

   a. global rating of adaptive functioning
   b. psychosocial and environmental problems
   c. general medical conditions that may be relevant to the patient's
      current behaviors or that may affect treatment
   d. familial communication style

4) Which would NOT be considered a limitation of a clinical interview?

   a. the information gathered is subjective and may be influenced or
      distorted by errors in memory or perception
   b. the person may be reluctant to directly share with the interviewer
      experiences that are embarrassing or socially undesirable
   c. interviews are expensive and time-consuming
   d. people may not be able to give a rational account of their problems due
      to the presence of limited verbal skills, a psychotic process, etc.

5) Analyzing a test on the basis of an explicit set of rules based on empirical research is referred to as what type of procedure?

   a. actuarial
   b. self report
   c. both sensitive and specific
   d. cookbook

6) A criticism of psychiatric diagnosis in the 1950's and 1960's was that:

   a. the diagnostic system in use was too detailed and included too many
      diagnostic categories
   b. the diagnostic system was too descriptive and did not make assumptions
      about etiology

c. once labelled with a diagnosis, individuals did not receive the appropriate treatment

d. once labelled with a diagnosis, an individual might be motivated to continue to act in a manner expected from someone who is mentally ill

7) Research on the physiological manifestations of marital dissatisfaction suggests that:

a. wives who do not express their negative emotions often display sleep difficulties

b. husbands who do not express their negative emotions often display changes in heart rate and skin conductance that indicate intense arousal

c. wives who verbally report negative emotion do not display any physiological changes

d. husbands who verbally express their negative emotions also show changes in their sleep patterns

8) When an observer is asked to make judgments about some aspect of an individual's behavior along a dimension, the observer would be using:

a. a projective instrument

b. a rating scale

c. a self-report inventory

d. a structured interview

9) Which of the following does NOT reflect a rationale for classifying abnormal behavior?

a. a diagnostic system can be used to help clinicians more effectively communicate with one another

b. a diagnostic system can be used to organize information that may be helpful for research purposes

c. a diagnostic system can be used to label people who are socially deviant

d. a diagnostic system can be used in making management and treatment decisions

10) Interpretation of a person's responses to the MMPI is based upon:

a. reviewing the clinical scale for which the person received the highest score

b. reading through all of the inventory items and noting how the person answered each one

c. reviewing the clinical scale for which the person received the lowest score

d. examining the pattern of scale scores, paying particular attention to those scales that have elevated scores

11) An example of a type of observational procedure would be:

   a. the Rorschach test
   b. the MMPI
   c. a behavioral coding system
   d. dynamic brain imaging

12) Which would NOT be considered a primary goal of assessment?

   a. making predictions
   b. reconstructing people's developmental history
   c. planning interventions
   d. evaluating interventions

13) An advantage of the MMPI is that:

   a. it provides information about the individual's test-taking attitude
   b. it assesses a wide range of problem areas that would take a clinician
      several hours to review in an interview
   c. it is scored objectively and is not influenced by the clinician's
      personal opinion about the individual taking the test
   d. all of the above

14) Which statement is TRUE regarding personality disorder diagnostic categories?

   a. two individuals must have the same combinations of diagnostic features
      in order to qualify for the same personality disorder diagnosis
   b. two individuals with different combinations of diagnostic features could
      qualify for the same personality disorder diagnosis
   c. an individual must have all of the features listed in the diagnostic
      criteria in order to qualify for a personality disorder diagnosis
   d. specific diagnostic criteria are given more weight in deciding whether
      or not an individual warrants the personality disorder diagnosis

15) How many axes are included in the DSM-IV?

   a. 3
   b. 4
   c. 5
   d. 6

16) What would be considered an advantage of a structured clinical interview compared to a regular clinical interview?

51

a. it provides the interviewer with a series of systematic questions that allow for the collection of important diagnostic information

b. it allows for the establishement of a better therapeutic rapport with the client

c. it allows the interviewer flexibility in gathering information

d. all of the above

17) Projective techniques place considerable emphasis upon which of the following?

a. the importance of unconscious motivations such as conflicts and impulses

b. the importance of familial values that may influence the person's behavior

c. the presence of symptoms, which suggest that the person has lost contact with reality and is presently psychotic

d. the importance of the person's cultural background in understanding his or her personality

18) An example of a measure that assesses a social system is:

a. Positron emission tomography

b. the Family Interaction Coding System

c. the Beck Depression Inventory

d. the Yale-Brown Obsessive-Compulsive Scale

19) Mary completed a depression scale and received a score of 24. The cut-off score for depression for this scale was 15, so Mary was classified as depressed. However, actually Mary was not really depressed but had a health problem that caused symptoms that overlapped with depressive symptoms. Mary would be considered:

a. a true positive

b. a false positive

c. a true negative

d. a false negative

20) Which type of study could be used to validate a clinical syndrome?

a. a follow-up study that demonstrated a distinctive course or outcome

b. a family study supporting that the syndrome "breeds true"

c. a study demonstrating an association between the clinical syndrome and an underlying biochemical abnormality

d. all of the above

21) An advantage of psychophysiological assessment is that:

a. these types of procedures do not depend on self-report and may be less likely to be under the person's control

b. physiological reactivity and stability is very consistent across people

c. physiological assessment is less expensive and less time consuming than the use of personality inventories

d. physiological procedures are frequently used in clinical settings

22) The most commonly used procedure in psychological assessment is:

a. self-report inventories
b. projective testing
c. clinical interview
d. behavioral observation

23) A limitation of brain-imaging procedures is that:

a. brain-imaging procedures can only be used with certain populations

b. although useful for research, brain-imaging procedures cannot be used for diagnostic purposes because norms have not yet been established

c. brain-imaging procedures tend to give imprecise information

d. the results of brain-imaging procedures tend to be overly responsive to outside factors such as whether the person is presently medicated

24) Which of the following problems could NOT be assessed through the use of an observational measure?

a. hand-washing
b. crying
c. low self-esteem
d. hitting, punching, or spitting at school

25) A limitation of the use of projective tests is:

a. information obtained from projective tests tends to duplicate what can already be obtained from a clinical interview

b. projective tests cannot be used with children

c. projective tests cannot be used with psychotic individuals

d. the reliability of scoring and interpretation appears to be low

26) Which type of study could be used to demonstrate the reliability of a set of diagnostic criteria?

a. a study demonstrating that clinicians using the same set of criteria

arrived at the same diagnosis for the same set of individuals
b. a study supporting that individuals with the same diagnosis responded to the same kind of treatment
c. a study supporting that the set of diagnostic criteria could be meaningful to other cultures when properly translated
d. all of the above

27) The L (Lie) Scale of the MMPI is an example of which type of scale?

a. reactivity
b. clinical
c. projective
d. validity

28) The probability that a person who has a positive test response will actually have the disorder is referred to as:

a. positive predictive power
b. negative predictive power
c. sensitivity
d. diagnostic power

29) The first two axes of the DSM-IV primarily focus on which of the following?

a. symptomatic behaviors
b. familial functioning
c. medical history
d. intrapsychic functioning

30) Which would NOT be considered a drawback of using a physiological assessment measure?

a. the equipment used may be intimidating to certain people
b. physiological responses can be influenced by many outside factors such as age and medication
c. physiological response measures have not demonstrated adequate validity
d. the stability of physiological response systems vary from person to person

BRIEF ESSAY

As a final exercise, write out answers to the following brief essay questions. Then compare your answers with the material presented in the text.

After you have answered these questions, review the "Critical Thinking" questions that are presented at the end of the text chapter. Answering these questions will help you integrate important issues and themes that have been featured throughout the chapter.

1. Briefly discuss the major assumptions of labeling theory. Then discuss your personal position about the theory; that is, to what extent do you agree with its major points?

2. Review examples of both scientific and nonscientific factors that affect the development of diagnostic systems. When do you see nonscientific factors playing an important role in this process?

3. Describe the major purposes of clinical assessment. What are the major assumptions regarding the nature of human behavior upon which the assessment process is based?

4. Pretend that you are a clinician who has just received a call from a potential client. The problem for which the client is seeking treatment is depression. What assessment procedures reviewed in your chapter could you use to determine whether or not the client is really depressed? What type of information would you expect to obtain from each method?

ANSWER KEY

MATCHING EXERCISES

1. s	11. o
2. g	12. e
3. q	13. r
4. d	14. j
5. n	15. m
6. t	16. h
7. i	17. a
8. l	18. k
9. c	19. p
10. f	20. b

MULTIPLE CHOICE EXERCISES

1. d	6. d	11. c
2. a	7. b	12. b
3. d	8. b	13. d
4. c	9. c	14. b
5. a	10. d	15. c

16. a	21. a	26. a
17. a	22. c	27. d
18. b	23. b	28. a
19. b	24. c	29. a
20. d	25. d	30. c

CHAPTER FIVE
MOOD DISORDERS

CHAPTER OUTLINE

Introduction to Mood Disorder
    Emotional Symptoms
    Cognitive Symptoms
        Suicidal Ideas
    Somatic Symptoms
    Other Problems Commonly Associated with Depression

Classification
    Brief Historical Perspective
    Contemporary Diagnostic Systems
        Unipolar Disorders
        Bipolar Disorders
    Course and Outcome
        Bipolar Disorders
        Unipolar Depression
    Incidence, Prevalence, and Morbid Risk
    Gender Differences
    Cross-cultural Differences
    Risk for Depression across the Life Span
    Epidemiology of Suicide

Etiological Considerations and Research
    Social Factors
        Freud's Theory of Depression
        The Impact of Loss and Stressful Life Events
            Stress as a Cause of Depression
            Depression as a Cause of Stress
    Psychological Factors
        Cognitive Responses to Failure and Disappointment
            Beck's Cognitive Model
            Hopelessness Theory
        Interpersonal Factors and Social Skills
            Lewinsohn's Behavioral Model
            Research on Interpersonal Factors
            Response Styles and Gender
        Integration of Cognitive and Interpersonal Factors
    Biological Factors
        Genetics
            Family Studies

                    Twin Studies
                    Combined Studies of Life Stress and Genetic Factors
                    Modes of Transmission and Linkage Studies
            Neurotransmitters and Depression
            The Neuroendocrine System
    The Interaction of Social, Psychological, and Biological Factors

    Psychological Interventions
            Cognitive Therapy
            Interpersonal Therapy
    Biological Interventions
            Electroconvulsive Therapy
            Antidepressant Medications
                    Tricyclics
                    Monoamine Oxidase Inhibitors
                    Selective Serotonin Reuptake Inhibitors
                    Lithium Carbonate
            Light Therapy for Seasonal Mood Disorders

Clinical Practice Guidelines

LEARNING OBJECTIVES

After reviewing the material presented in this chapter, you should be able to:

*   distinguish clinical depression from a depresssed mood

*   define emotion, affect, mood, depression, and mania

*   contrast major depressive disorder with dysthymia

*   distinguish bipolar I, bipolar II, and cyclothymia

*   know the average age of onset for depression and bipolar disorder, as well
        as the typical recovery rates for each disorder

*   understand how social factors, especially interpersonal loss, can be
        influential in the development of depression

*   contrast Beck's cognitive model with the Abramson/Alloy hopelessness model
        of depression

*   appreciate the interaction between social, psychological, and biological

58

factors in the development and maintenance maintenance of mood disorders

* compare interpersonal therapy with cognitive therapy approaches

* understand the pros and cons of electroconvulsive shock therapy

KEY TERMS AND CONCEPTS

Following is a list of key terms and concepts that are featured in the chapter and are important for you to know. Write out the definitions of each of these terms and check your answers with the definitions in the text.

Emotion
Affect
Mood
Depression
Mania
Mood disorders
Unipolar mood disorder
Bipolar mood disorder
Double depression
Dysphoric mood
Euphoria
Somatic symptoms
Psychomotor retardation
Comorbidity
Hypomania
Cyclothymia
Melancholia
Point prevalence
Seasonal affective disorder
Ambivalence
Cognitive theory of depression
Schema model
Hopelessness theory
Learned helplessness theory
Vulnerability
Familial pattern of transmission
Proband
Linkage studies
Catecholamine hypothesis of depression
Indolamine hypothesis of depression

Hypothalamic-pituitary-adrenal axis
Tricyclics
Monoamine oxidase inhibitors
Selective serotonin reuptake inhibitors
Dexamethasone suppression test

KEY NAMES

The following individuals have made important contributions to the material presented in the chapter. Write out the names of these individuals and the theories, research, or treatments with which they are associated. Then check your answers with the information in your text.

Edwin Schneidman
Emil Kraeplin
Adolf Meyer
Arthur Kleinman
Sigmund Freud
George Brown
Aaron Beck
Lynn Abramson
Lauren Alloy
Martin Seligman
Peter Lewinsohn
James Coyne
Susan Nolan-Hoeksema
Ian Gotlib
Constance Hammen
Jay Weiss

MATCHING QUESTIONS

Match the following terms and names with the definitions presented below. The answers can be found at the end of this chapter.

a.	unipolar mood disorder	k.	interpersonal therapy
b.	double depression	l.	proband
c.	euphoria	m.	catecholamine hypothesis
d.	depressive triad	n.	analogue study
e.	dysthymia	o.	Kraeplin
f.	Beck	p.	locus
g.	cyclothymia	q.	comorbidity

60

h.   HPA axis
i.   tricyclics
j.   point prevalence

r.   lithium carbonate
s.   Lewinsohn
t.   cognitive
      therapy for depression

1) ____   focus on the most negative features on one's self, one's environment, and one's future

2) ____   an influential psychologist who developed a behavioral model of depression

3) ____   a type of experiment which focuses on behaviors of interest that occur in the natural environment

4) ____   person experiences only episodes of depression

5) ____   assists patients in developing a better understanding of their current, close relationships and the interpersonal issues that may contribute to their depression

6) ____   an influential figure proposing a cognitive theory of depression

7) ____   drugs that block the uptake of specific neurotransmitters from the synapse

8) ____   an individual in a family study who has been diagnosed as having a particular disorder

9) ____   an effective form of treatment for manic episodes

10) ____   an episode of severe depression which occurs during an episode of chronic mild depression

11) ____   a gene at a particular location

12) ____   chronic mild depression persisting for several years

13) ____   a less severe form of bipolar disorder

14) ____   a theory of depression that focused on decreased levels of certain chemicals in the brain

15) ____   simultaneous manifestation of two disorders or syndromes

16) _____ a feeling of extreme joy, optimism, and cheerfulness

17) _____ an important pathway in the endocrine system that may contribute to vulnerability to mood disorders

18) _____ physician who divided the major forms of mental disorder into two categories: dementia praecox and manic-depressive psychosis

19) _____ assisting patients to replace self-defeating cognitions with more objective and rational self-statements

20) _____ percentage of the population that reports certain experiences at a given point in time

MULTIPLE CHOICE QUESTIONS

The following multiple choice questions will test your comprehension of the material presented in the chapter. Circle the correct choice for each question in the section. Then compare your answers with those at the end of the chapter.

1) Which of the following is NOT a general area describing the signs and symptoms representative of mood disorders?

    a. emotional symptoms
    b. psychological symptoms
    c. somatic symptoms
    d. cognitive symptoms

2) A promising form of treatment for seasonal affective disorder is:

    a. light therapy
    b. lithium carbonate
    c. nutritional therapy
    d. meditation

3) What is the percent of completed suicides that occur as a result of a primary mood disorder?

    a. 15 - 22%
    b. 35 - 44%
    c. 50 - 67%
    d. 78 - 90%

4) Which is an example of a somatic symptom?

    a. suicidal ideation
    b. loss of interest
    c. sleep disturbance
    d. low self-esteem

5) An advantage of an analogue study is that:

    a. experimental procedures may be employed
    b. it is easy to generalize the results beyond the laboratory
    c. human subjects are not used
    d. it is easy to reproduce a clinical disorder in the laboratory

6) Which symptom would NOT be considered diagnostic for clinical depression?

    a. racing thoughts
    b. fatigue or loss of energy
    c. feelings of worthlessness
    d. difficulty concentrating

7) Why might it be more difficult to diagnose depression in the elderly?

    a. cognitive impairment or other problems common in the elderly may mask the symptoms of depression
    b. the elderly are more reluctant to seek treatment for depression
    c. the symptoms and features of depression change as age increases
    d. the elderly are less likely to report somatic symptoms associated with depression

8) Results from the Treatment of Depresssion Collaborative Research Program indicate that:

    a. both types of psychological treatment (interpersonal and cognitive) were as effective as antidepressant medication
    b. patients who received interpersonal therapy did not show gains with cognitive problems
    c. placebo was equally effective to antidepressant medication
    d. cognitive therapy was superior to interpersonal therapy in its effectiveness

9) Which age group has experienced increased rates of suicide since the 1960s?

a. adolescents
b. people who are thirty-something
c. people between the ages of 45 - 55
d. people over 65

10) When two loci occupy positions that are close together on the same chromosome they are said to be:

a. polygenic
b. matched
c. homogenous
d. linked

11) Which is an example of a social factor which may contribute to the onset of depression?

a. the belief that one cannot control events in one's life
b. cognitive distortions
c. stressful life events
d. neuroendocrine disturbances

12) Which disorder is often comorbid with a mood disorder?

a. schizophrenia
b. dissociative disorder
c. paranoid personality disorder
d. alcoholism

13) Which is a fundamental assumption about Freud's theory of depression?

a. depressed people are not able to experience guilt
b. depression is an extension of the normal process of grieving
c. depressed people do not depend on others to maintain their self-esteem
d. depressed people are really angry with someone else

14) What age would an individual most likely experience a first episode of bipolar mood disorder?

a. 18 - 23 years
b. 28 - 33 years
c. 38 - 43 years
d. 48 - 53 years

15) Which of the following is a common element of suicide?
   a. the common goal of suicide is cessation of consciousness
   b. the common emotion in suicide is anger
   c. the common purpose of suicide is to get revenge
   d. the common stressor in suicide is financial difficulties

16) Which of the following is NOT a factor which has been found to increase vulnerability to depression in women?

   a. loss of mother at an early age
   b. lack of employment away from the home
   c. children leaving the home for educational and professional pursuits
   d. lack of an intimate, confiding relationship

17) Decreased need for sleep, pressure to keep talking, grandiosity, and distractibility are common symptoms of which disorder?

   a. mania
   b. dysthymia
   c. double depression
   d. cyclothymia

18) Advantages of selective serotonin reuptake inhibitors include all BUT which of the following?

   a. fewer side effects
   b. less likely to have multiple episodes of depression
   c. less dangerous in the case of an overdose
   d. easier for the patient to take

19) Which is an example of a depressogenic premise?

   a. "I find time in my day to relax"
   b. "I should be at the top of my performance at all times"
   c. "I congratulate myself when I finish a hard day at work"
   d. "I try to forgive myself when I screw things up"

20) Research on electroconvulsive therapy supports that:

   a. memory impairment may be permanent
   b. only bipolar depressed patients respond to ECT
   c. ECT is as effective as placebo
   d. some depressed patients may respond to ECT more than to antidepressant medication

21) Which statement is NOT true about unipolar depression?

    a. episodes of unipolar depression tend to be longer in duration, compared to episodes of depression in bipolar disorder
    b. at least half of unipolar patients will experience more than one episode
    c. female patients tend to relapse more quickly than male patients
    d. unipolar patients have their first episode of depression at a much younger age than do bipolar patients

22) Some depressed people exhibit a depressogenic attributional style that is characterized by the tendency to explain negative events in terms of:

    a. internal, stable, global factors
    b. internal, unstable, specific factors
    c. external, unstable, specific factors
    d. external, stable, specific factors

23) A standard part of cognitive treatment for depression would be:

    a. gaining insight into suppressed anger in close relationships
    b. developing a better understanding of family relationships
    c. substituting more flexible self-statements for rigid and absolute ones
    d. nondirect discussions of unexpressed emotions

24) An important assumption of the hopelessness theory of depression is:

    a. loss of a parent early in life increases risk for depression
    b. desirable events will not occur regardless of what the person does
    c. depressed people are more likely to feel in control of the events of their lives
    d. depressed people have a positive impact on other people's moods

25) Which type of coping behavior is associated with longer and more severely depressed moods?

    a. processing style
    b. ruminative style
    c. intellectual style
    d. distracting style

26) Which of the following is NOT indicated by the Clinical Practice Guidelines for treatement of Depression?

a. antidepressant medication

b. psychotherapy (cognitive, behavioral, or interpersonal)

c. antidepressant medication combined with psychotherapy

d. cognitive psychotherapy combined with interpersonal psychotherapy

27) Studies investigating genetic transmission of mood disorders indicate that:

a. the genetic factors are more influential in bipolar disorders than major depressive disorder

b. the concordance rate for mood disorders is higher for DZ than MZ twins

c. there is no increased risk for bipolar disorder for relatives of bipolar

d. genetic factors account for about 90% of the variance for dysthymia

28) Which statement is true regarding the impact of stressful life events on depression?

a. positive events like holidays may precipitate depressive episodes

b. events that involve major losses of important people or roles may precipitate depressive episodes

c. events that are within a person's control are most likely to precipitate depressive episodes

d. depressed persons experience lower numbers of stressful events prior to the onset of their depressive episodes compared to family members

29) How do depressed people often respond to a test dose of dexamethasone?

a. they show a suppression of cortisol secretion

b. they show a failure of suppression of cortisol secretion

c. they show a dramatic increase of cortisol secretion

d. they show an abnormal fluctuation of cortisol secretion

30) An example of a DSM-IV subtype of depression is:

a. retarded

b. dysphoric

c. narcisstic

d. melancholic

BRIEF ESSAY

As a final exercise, write out answers to the following brief essay questions. Then compare your answers with the material presented in the text.

After you have answered these questions, review the "Critical Thinking" questions that are presented at the end of the text chapter. Answering these questions will help you integrate important issues and themes that have been featured throughout the chapter.

1. What are the primary issues that have been at the center of the controversy about definitions of mood disorders? Would you advocate the use of subtyping in mood disorders? Why?

2. Discuss the methodological problems that one encounters in studying mood disorder across cultures. How have cross-cultural investigations assisted our understanding of mood disorders?

3. Describe the model of depression that emphasizes the interplay between cognitive and interpersonal factors.

ANSWER KEY

MATCHING EXERCISES

1. d	11. p
2. s	12. e
3. n	13. g
4. a	14. m
5. k	15. q
6. f	16. c
7. i	17. h
8. l	18. o
9. r	19. t
10. b	20. j

MULTIPLE CHOICE EXERCISES

1. b	6. a	11. c
2. a	7. a	12. d
3. c	8. a	13. d
4. c	9. a	14. b
5. a	10. d	15. a
16. c	21. d	26. d
17. a	22. a	27. a
18. b	23. c	28. b
19. b	24. b	29. b
20. d	25. b	30. d

CHAPTER SIX
ANXIETY DISORDERS

CHAPTER OUTLINE

Overview

Typical Symptoms and Associated Features
    Anxiety
    Panic Attacks
    Phobias
        Agoraphobia
    Obsessions and Compulsions
    Other Disorders Commonly Associated with Anxiety

Classification
    Brief Historical Perspective
    Subclassification
    Contemporary Diagnostic Systems (DSM-IV)

Epidemiology
    Incidence, Prevalence, and Morbid Risk
    Gender Differences
    Cross-cultural Comparisons

Etiological Considerations and Research
    Social Factors
        Psychoanalytic Theory
        Developmental Precursors: Separation Anxiety
        Stressful Life Events
    Psychological Factors
        Learning Processes: Specific Phobias
            Seligman's Preparedness Model
            Vicarious Learning and Preparedness
        Cognitive Factors
            Perception of Control: Panic Attacks
            Catastrophic Misinterpretation: Panic Attacks
            Worrying: Generalized Anxiety Disorder
            Thought Suppression: Obsessive-Compulsive Disorder
        Interpersonal Factors: Social Phobias
    Biological Factors
        Twin Studies
        Pharmacological Provocation of Panic
            False Suffocation Alarm Theory

Treatment
    Psychological Interventions
        Exposure: Desensitization and Flooding
        Prolonged Exposure and Response Prevention
        Applied Relaxation
        Cognitive Therapy
    Biological Interventions
        Antianxiety Medications
        Tricyclic Antidepressants
        MAO Inhibitors
        Selective Serotonin Reuptake Inhibitors
        General Recommendations

LEARNING OBJECTIVES

After reviewing the material presented in this chapter, you should be able to:

*   contrast anxiety with fear; define anxiety

*   name some of the key physical and cognitive symptoms involved in panic attacks

*   compare specific phobias with agoraphobia

*   define obsessions and compulsions

*   understand the historical development of the term anxiety disorder from terms like psychasthenia, neurosis, and hysteria

*   rank the prevalence rates of the anxiety disorders in order

*   understand the basic classification system that DSM-IV uses for panic disorder, specific phobia, social phobia, generalized anxiety disorder, obsessive-compulsive disorder, and agoraphobia

*   compare the psychoanalytic theory of anxiety, in which repression plays a crucial role, to the approach of Ainsworth and Bowlby, in which early attachment plays the key role in determining anxiety

*   understand Seligman's preparedness model in explaining why certain phobias are "easier" to develop

*   name three cognitive factors that are considered influential in the development of anxiety disorders

*   describe the results of family studies and twin studies of incidence of anxiety disorders

*   appreciate the differences between systematic desensitization and flooding in treatment of phobias

*   describe the advantages and disadvantages of using benzodiazepines and tricyclics in the treatment of various anxiety disorders

KEY TERMS AND CONCEPTS

Following is a list of key terms and concepts that are featured in the chapter and are important for you to know. Write out the definitions of each of these terms and check your answers with the definitions in the text.

Fear
Anxiety
Anxious apprehension
Negative affect
Positive affect
Panic attack
Phobia
Agoraphobia
Obsessions
Compulsions
Psychasthenia
Neurosis
Generalized anxiety disorder
Specific phobia
Social phobia
Mixed anxiety-depressive disorder
Kayak angst
Signal anxiety
Attachment theory
Preparedness theory
Vicarious learning
Experimental neurosis
Worry
Thought suppression
Desensitization

Flooding
Imaginal exposure
In vivo exposure
Statistical significance
Clinical importance
Decatastrophizing
Benzodiazepines
Gamma-aminobutyric acid (GABA)
Tricyclic antidepressants
MAO inhibitors
Selective serotonin reuptake inhibitors

KEY NAMES

The following individuals have made important contributions to the material presented in the chapter. Write out the names of these individuals and the theories, research, or treatment with which they are associated. Then check your answers with the information in your text.

Sigmund Freud
Pierre Janet
Mary Ainsworth
John Bowlby
Martin Seligman
Susan Mineka
David Clark
Thomas Borkovec
Kenneth Kendler
Donald Klein

MATCHING QUESTIONS

Match the following terms and names with the definitions presented below. The answers can be found at the end of the chapter.

a. lactate infusion
b. compulsions
c. attachment theory
d. social phobia
e. flooding
f. signal anxiety
g. decatastrophizing
h. panic attack

k. agoraphobia
l. psychasthenia
m. response prevention
n. preparedness theory
o. anxious apprehension
p. obsessions
q. Donald Klein
r. specific phobia

i. mixed anxiety-depression
j. desensitization hierarchy

s. thought suppression
t. Martin Seligman

1) _____ a newly proposed category of anxiety disorder that includes symptoms of both anxiety and depression

2) _____ an exaggerated fear of being in situations from which escape may be difficult

3) _____ maladaptive anxiety response which includes the experience of negative emotion, a focus on the self, and a sense of uncontrollability

4) _____ a sudden, overwhelming experience of terror or fright, accompanied by a range of physical sensations

5) _____ repetitive, unwanted, and intrusive cognitive events that may be experienced as images or impulses

6) _____ an active attempt to stop thinking about something

7) _____ a marked and persistent unreasonable fear that is cued by the presence or anticipation of a specific object or situation

8) _____ a researcher who has developed an integrated model of panic attacks and agoraphobia incorporating both psychological and biological factors

9) _____ proposes that organisms are biologically prepared, on the basis of neural pathways, to learn certain types of associations

10) _____ repetitive behaviors which are considered irrational by the person who performs them

11) _____ a psychologist who has proposed that humans are prepared to develop intense, persistent fears only to a select group of objects

12) _____ a diagnostic term introduced by Pierre Janet that included many different symptoms associated with anxiety

13) _____ proposes that humans are prepared to develop strong attachments to their caretakers

14) _____ a laboratory procedure which has been found to provoke a panic attack

73

in patients with a history of anxiety disorders

15) _____   an excessive or unreasonable fear of performing a particular act in front of other people, leading to avoidance of that situation

16) _____   a technique whereby a patient is not allowed to perform the compulsive ritual which may temporarily reduce anxiety

17) _____   indicates that an instinctual impulse previously associated with punishment and disapproval is about to be acted upon

18) _____   an ordered list of feared stimuli, beginning with those items provoking only small amounts of fear, and progressing through stimuli that are increasingly feared

19) _____   a therapeutic technique whereby a patient is immediately exposed to stimuli most frightening to him or her

20) _____   a cognitive technique in which the patient is asked to imagine a worst case scenario, followed by careful analysis of possible distortions in thinking

MULTIPLE CHOICE QUESTIONS

The following multiple choice questions will test your comprehension of the material presented in the chapter. Circle the correct choice for each question in the section. Then compare your answers with those at the end of the chapter.

1) The most frequently used types of minor tranquilizers for the treatment of anxiety disorders are:

     a. tricyclics
     b. benzodiazapines
     c. serotonin
     d. GABA inhibitors

2) Which of the following is LEAST likely to be present in an anxiety disorder?

     a. lack of insight
     b. social impairment
     c. significant personal distress
     d. negative emotional response

3) Which of the following is an example of a potential unconditioned stimulus (UCS) which could contribute to the development of a phobia?

    a. loss of a relationship
    b. chronic occupational difficulties
    c. a painfully loud and unexpected noise
    d. a sad song

4) _____ is experienced in the face of real and immediate danger, _____ is a diffuse emotional reaction that is out or proportion to threats from the environment.

    a. anxiety, fear
    b. worry, anxiety
    c. fear, anxiety
    d. worry, fear

5) The results of family studies investigating transmission of anxiety disorders support that:

    a. there appears to be no genetic component to OCD
    b. social phobia is the most inheritable form of anxiety disorder
    c. panic disorder and generalized anxiety disorder are etiologically
       separate disorders
    d. the most inheritable anxiety disorder is specific phobia

6) The two most common types of compulsions are:

    a. counting and repeating
    b. cleaning and checking
    c. sorting and counting
    d. checking and writing

7) A junior in college, Sam is acutely distressed at the thought of having to write in front of other people. He is afraid that he will drop his pen, lose control of his writing, or do something else embarassing while other people are watching him. While he is able to write in the privacy of his room, this fear has impaired his ability to take notes in classes. His most likely diagnosis would be:

    a. specific phobia
    b. agoraphobia
    c. generalized anxiety disorder
    d. social phobia

8) The discovery of laboratory procedures that reliably induce panic attacks is important because:

    a. they offer investigators the opportunity to research the antecedents and consequences of panic attacks
    b. brain activities that occur during a panic attack may be monitored
    c. such procedures may be fruitful in developing a map of the specific areas of the brain that mediate anxiety symptoms
    d. all of the above

9) Which of the following is the most common type of abnormal behavior?

    a. phobias
    b. major depression
    c. generalized anxiety disorder
    d. dysthymia

10) Specific phobias may be best understood in terms of learning experiences. The association between the object and intense fear can develop through all BUT which of the following?

    a. direct experience
    b. observational learning
    c. exposure to fear-irrelevant stimuli
    d. exposure to warnings and instructions about dangerous situations

11) Which statement is TRUE regarding the relationship between anxiety and other disorders?

    a. substance dependence is rarely associated with anxiety disorders
    b. anxiety disorders overlap considerably with other anxiety disorders
    c. anxiety disorders overlap considerably with dissociative disorders
    d. anxiety disorders do not appear to be associated with depressive disorders

12) "Free-floating" anxiety would be most characteristic of which anxiety disorder?

    a. social phobia
    b. panic disorder
    c. obsessive-compulsive disorder
    d. generalized anxiety disorder

13) Which of the following statements would NOT be consistent with Freud's later version of anxiety?

    a. repression is the product of anxiety
    b. anxiety is the result of a harsh superego in conflict with the defense
       mechanisms that are employed by the ego
    c. the specific form of overt symptoms is determined by the defense
       mechanisms that are employed by the ego
    d. different types of anxiety disorders can be distinguished by many
       factors within the analytic framework, for example, the developmental
       stage at which the person experiences problems

14) Anxiety disorder categories did not emerge in psychiatric classifications during the last century primarily because:

    a. the prevalence of anxiety disorders was much lower during the last
       century
    b. they were considered to be neurological disorders
    c. very few cases of anxiety disorders required institutionalization
    d. physicians were not trained to recognize the symptoms of anxiety
       disorders

15) Which of the following is NOT a symptom of a panic attack?

    a. feeling of choking
    b. trembling
    c. nausea
    d. headache

16) According to attachment theory:

    a. individual differences in attachment styles, presumably influenced by
       early social relationships, may contribute to the development of future
       anxiety reactions
    b. securely attached infants are the least likely to protest when their
       caretaker leaves the room
    c. humans are prepared to develop weak attachments to their caretakers to
       foster individual independence
    d. all of the above

17) Research on the relationship between stressful life events and anxiety disorders suggests that:

    a. the onset of agoraphobia may be associated with interpersonal conflict

b. marital distress is associated with the onset of simple phobia

c. the onset of agoraphobia may be associated with the experience of a conditioning event, such as a sudden painful injury

d. severe loss is associated with the onset of an anxiety disorder

18) Which of the following cognitive factors appears to share an important relationship with panic attacks?

a. perception of control over events in one's environment

b. thought suppression

c. cognitive minimization of traumatic events

d. all-or-none thinking about future events

19) Which of the following is NOT included in the DSM-IV's classification of anxiety disorders?

a. panic disorder

b. agoraphobia

c. cyclothymia

d. obsessive-compulsive disorder

20) If a panic attack only occurs in the presence of a particular stimulus, it is said to be:

a. a situationally cued attack

b. an anticipated attack

c. a "below threshold" attack

d. a cognitively processed attack

21) Karen has consistent worries that she is going to lose her job, that something is going to happen to her husband and that she will be alone, and that her health may take a turn for the worse. She knows that her worries are causing friction in her marital relationship, but she feels that she cannot control these thoughts, although she repeatedly tries to put them out of her mind. Although she has always been a "worrier", the intensity and frequency of her worries has gotten worse in the past year. Karen's most likely diagnosis would be:

a. agoraphobia

b. panic disorder

c. generalized anxiety disorder

d. simple phobia

22) The most serious adverse side effects of benzodiazepines is:

a. heart palpitations

b. significant weight gain

c. the dietary restrictions which patients must observe while using them

d. their potential for addiction

23) The types of symptoms most characteristic of a panic attack are:

    a. interpersonal difficulties

    b. physical sensations

    c. emotional reactions

    d. cognitive reactions

24) Cross-cultural research on anxiety disorders suggests that:

    a. anxiety disorders are not experienced in certain cultures

    b. phobic avoidance is the most commonly reported symptom across cultures

    c. the focus of typical anxiety complaints can vary dramatically across cultures

    d. anxiety disorders are more common in preliterate cultures

25) An important consideration in diagnosing panic disorder is:

    a. the person must experience recurrent, situationally cued panic attacks

    b. the person must experience recurrent panic attacks in anticipation of a feared event

    c. the person must report the experience of feeling out of control

    d. the person must experience recurrent unexpected panic attacks

26) Which of the following is NOT included in the DSM-IV as criteria to establish the boundary between normal behavior and compulsive rituals?

    a. the rituals cause marked distress

    b. the rituals can be observed by other people

    c. the rituals interfere with normal occupational and social functioning

    d. the rituals take more than one hour per day to perform

27) Which of the following would be a typical situation that would cause problems for an agoraphobic?

    a. travelling on the subway

    b. speaking to a friend on the phone

    c. cleaning the house

    d. encountering a snake

28) According to recent research, what percent of the people who qualify for an anxiety disorder diagnosis actually seek treatment for their disorder?

   a. 15%
   b. 25%
   c. 40%
   d. 50%

29) What is an important difference between compulsions and some addictive behaviors such as gambling?

   a. addictive behaviors reduce anxiety more effectively than compulsions
   b. compulsions are more resistant to treatment
   c. addictive behaviors are not repetitive in nature
   d. compulsions reduce anxiety but they do not produce pleasure

30) Women are about twice as likely as men to experience all BUT which of the following anxiety disorders?

   a. social phobia
   b. agoraphobia
   c. specific phobia
   d. panic disorder

BRIEF ESSAY

As a final exercise, write out answers to the following brief essay questions. Then compare your answers with the material presented in the text.

After you have answered these questions, review the "Critical Thinking" questions that are presented at the end of the text chapter. Answering these questions will help you integrate important issues and themes that have been featured throughout the chapter.

1. Learning processes have been theoretically associated with the development of phobias, while cognitive factors have been used to explain the development of panic attacks. Review the prominent learning and cognitive theories that account for each type of disorder. Do you think that differences in etiological processes imply that these disorders are really unrelated? Why or why not?

2. Discuss the overlap between anxiety and depression. Do you think that anxiety and depression are separate types of disorders, or do you think that they represent different manifestations of the same problem? What evidence supports your position?

3. Consider the following psychological interventions used for the treatment of anxiety disorders: desensitization, flooding, prolonged exposure and response prevention, and cognitive therapy. Select an anxiety disorder and discuss how you would approach treatment for this disorder. Which intervention techniques(s) would you choose and why?

4. False suffocation alarm theory is a theoretical model of panic attacks and agoraphobia that integrates biological and psychological factors. Discuss this theory, highlighting both the main assumptions of the model and the research findings which support these assumptions.

ANSWER KEY

MATCHING EXERCISES

1. i	11. t
2. k	12. l
3. o	13. c
4. h	14. a
5. p	15. d
6. s	16. m
7. r	17. f
8. q	18. j
9. n	19. e
10. b	20. g

MULTIPLE CHOICE EXERCISES

1. b	6. b	11. b
2. a	7. d	12. d
3. c	8. d	13. b
4. c	9. a	14. c
5. c	10. c	15. d

16. a	21. c	26. b
17. a	22. d	27. a
18. a	23. b	28. b
19. c	24. c	29. d
20. a	25. d	30. a

CHAPTER SEVEN
MALADAPTIVE RESPONSES TO STRESS

CHAPTER OUTLINE

Stress: An overview
    Defining stress, stressors, distress, and stress response
        Stress as a stimulus
        Stress as a stimulus and a response
    Typical symptoms and associated features of stress
        Physiological responses to stress
        General adaptation syndrome
            Different physiological responses to different
            stressors
        Emotional responses to stress
        Cognitive responses to stress
        Behavioral responses to stress
        Illness as a cause of stress
    Classification of maladaptive responses to stress
        Brief historical perspective
        Contemporary approaches
        Stress and psychological disorders

Cardiovascular disease
    Typical symptoms and associated features of hypertension and
    coronary heart disease
    Subclassification and epidemiology
        Epidemiology of cardiovascular disorder
            Epidemiology of coronary heart disease
            Epidemiology of hypertension
    Etiological considerations and research on cardiovascular disease
        Psychological factors in cardiovascular disease
            Physiological reactivity to stress
            Life stressors and cardiovascular disease
            Type A behavior and styles of responding to
            stressors
        Social factors in cardiovascular disease
        Integrating biological, psychological, and social risk
        factors
    Prevention and treatment of cardiovascular disease
        Primary prevention
        Secondary prevention
        Tertiary prevention or treatment

Post traumatic stress disorder (PTSD)
     Typical symptoms and associated features of PTSD
     Subclassification and epidemiology
          Epidemiology of PTSD
     Ecological considerations and research on PTSD
          Biological factors in PTSD
               Biological effects of exposure to trauma
          Psychological factors in PTSD
          Social factors in PTSD
     Treatment of PTSD
          Emergency treatment of trauma victims and prevention
          of PTSD
          Treatment of PTSD
          Course and outcome

Summary

LEARNING OBJECTIVES

After reviewing the material presented in this chapter, you should be able to:

*   define stress, stressors, and the stress response

*   understand what is meant by the emergency reaction and the general
        adaptation syndrome

*   distinguish psychosomatic disorders from somatoform disorders

*   compare the symptoms of hypertension to those of coronary heart disease

*   describe what the specificity hypothesis is and why it is currently rejected

*   distinguish primary and secondary hypertension

*   understand the impact of low control, high demand job strain on hypertension

*   describe the major characteristics of the Type A personality

*   define and list the DSM-IV symptoms of Post Traumatic Stress Disorder

*   distinguish PTSD from acute stress disorder and adjustment disorder

*   describe some of the treatment approaches utilized with victims of PTSD

KEY TERMS AND CONCEPTS

Following is a list of key terms and concepts that are featured in the chapter and are important for you to know. Write out the definitions of each of these terms and check your answers with the definitions in the text.

Stress
Traumatic stress
Posttraumatic stress disorder (PTSD)
Behavioral medicine
Health psychology
Stressor
Distress
Stress response
Life change units
Life transitions
Emergency response
Fight or flight
General adaptation syndrome (GAS)
Stage of alarm
Stage of resistance
Exhaustion
Psychoneuroimmunology
Glucocorticoids
T cells
Lymphocytes
Mitogens
Immunosuppression
Physiological toughness
Problem-focused coping
Emotion-focused coping
Health behavior
Illness behavior
Social support
Psychosomatic disorder
Somatoform disorders
Factitious disorder
Germ theory
Psychosomatic
Specificity hypothesis
Adjustment disorders
Cardiovascular disease (CVD)
Hypertension

Coronary heart disease (CHD)
Myocardial infarction (MI)
Systolic blood pressure
Diastolic blood pressure
Angina pectoris
Sudden cardiac death (SCD)
Secondary hypertension
Essential hypertension
Atherosclerosis
Coronary occlusion
Myocardial ischemia
Physiological reactivity
Type A behavior pattern
Longitudinal study
Cross-sectional approach
Social ecology
Antihypertensives
Beta blockers
Stress management
Biofeedback
Role playing
Flashbacks
Dissociative state
Victimization
Acute stress disorder
Two-factor theory
Rape crisis center
Trauma desensitization

KEY NAMES

The following individuals have made important contributions to the material presented in the chapter. Write out the names of these individuals and the theories, research, or treatment with which they are associated. Then check your answers with the information in your text.

Richard Lazarus
Hans Selye
Walter Cannon
Hippocrates
Louis Pasteur
Franz Alexander
Meyer Friedman
Ray Rosenman

MATCHING QUESTIONS

Match the following terms and names with the definitions presented below. The answers can be found at the end of the chapter.

a. traumatic stress
b. stage of resistance
c. problem-focused coping
d. Richard Lazarus
e. hypertension
f. psychosomatic
g. type A behavior pattern
h. coronary occlusion
i. acute stress disorder
j. Hans Selye

k. Franz Alexander
l. sudden cardiac death (SCD)
m. cardiovascular disease (CVD)
n. adjustment disorder
o. Walter Cannon
p. myocardial infarction (MI)
q. stressor
r. stage of exhaustion
s. emotion-focused coping
t. atherosclerosis

1) _____ Selye identified this as the mechanism through which stress causes physical illness

2) _____ involves exposure to some catastrophic event that is outside the realm of normal human experience

3) _____ coined by Heinroth in 1818, this is a way to emphasize that both mind and body are important in the development of disease

4) _____ an attempt to alter internal distress, perhaps because it is impossible to control the stressor itself

5) _____ usually defined as death within 24 hours of a coronary episode

6) _____ maintained that physical or psychological threats produce generalized emotional reactions accompanied by psycho-physiological responses

7) _____ a group of disorders that affect the heart and circulatory system

8) _____ the thickening of the coronary artery wall that occurs over age as a result of the accumulation of blood lipids (fats)

9) _____ characterized by a somewhat less intense reaction to trauma that lasts less than 4 weeks

10) _____ this is commonly known as a heart attack

86

11) _____ an example of this might be ending a relationship with a significant other because it is causing problems

12) _____ a trying event or stimulus irrespective of its effect on the individual

13) _____ not considered to be a mental disorder, this is caused by normal stress and involves normal emotional, cognitive, and behavioral reactions

14) _____ argued that stress arises not from life events themselves but from the individual's cognitive appraisal of these events

15) _____ results either from arteries that are completely blocked by fatty deposits or from blood clots that make their way to the heart muscle

16) _____ a period of replenishment during which the body becomes physiologically prepared to deal with new threats

17) _____ a characterological response to challenge that is competitive, urgent, hostile, impatient, and achievement-striving

18) _____ often referred to as the "silent killer," this is also commonly known as high blood pressure

19) _____ consistent with the specificity hypothesis, he attempted to classify physical illnesses according to personality type

20) _____ he defined stress in terms of a combination of a trying event and a reaction to the event

MULTIPLE CHOICE QUESTIONS

The following multiple choice questions will test your comprehension of the material presented in the chapter. Circle the correct choice for each question in the section. Then compare your answers with those at the end of the chapter.

1) All of the following are criticisms of the Holmes and Rahe Social Re-Adjustment Rating Scale EXCEPT:

   a. the inclusion of both positive and negative events as stressors
   b. failure to distinguish between transient and chronic life events
   c. a given stressor does not always produce the same number of life change units for all individuals in all situations

d. all of the above are criticisms of this scale

2) Generally, hypertension is defined by a systolic blood pressure of above _____ and a diastolic blood pressure of above _____.

    a. 110; 60
    b. 120; 70
    c. 130; 80
    d. 140; 90

3) According to Walter Cannon, _____ is the mobilization of the body in reaction to a perceived threat.

    a. stage of alarm
    b. generalized arousal
    c. emergency response
    d. physiological toughness

4) Many people who suffer from PTSD also meet the diagnostic criteria for another mental disorder, particularly _____ and _____.

    a. depression; substance abuse
    b. hypomania; antisocial personality disorder
    c. depression; adjustment disorder
    d. hypomania; paranoid personality disorder

5) All of the following are cultural myths of sexual assault EXCEPT:

    a. women who are raped provoke it
    b. women who are raped are "damaged goods"
    c. women who are raped often enjoy it
    d. most women who are raped are raped by an acquaintance

6) Although somewhat stressful, _____ decreases negative responding to an actual stressor.

    a. predictability
    b. anticipation
    c. control
    d. appraisal

7) Anxiety, depression, and _____ are considered to be the primary affective responses to stressors.

a. anger
b. tension
c. an upset stomach
d. aggression

8) Stress plays a role in:

a. all physical disorders
b. all psychological disorders
c. both a and b
d. none of the above

9) _____ of all deaths from CHD occur within 24 hours of a coronary event.

a. one-quarter
b. one-half
c. one-third
d. two-thirds

10) Jack, who is a Vietnam Veteran, tries to run for cover every time he hears an airplane pass by overhead. Jack's reaction to the airplane can best be described as a:

a. flashback
b. dissociative state
c. brief psychotic reaction
d. hallucination

11) This term is used to describe people who habitually and deliberately pretend to have a physical illness.

a. hypochondriasis
b. psychosis
c. factitious disorder
d. adjustment disorder

12) Which of the following would most likely have the greatest risk for suffering from high blood pressure?

a. African-American male who is homeless
b. White male who is a stock broker
c. African-American female who is an attorney
d. White female who is a homemaker

13) According to one study conducted in the St. Louis area, the most common cause of PTSD among men was:

    a. observing domestic violence in the home as a child
    b. being a victim of physical abuse as a child
    c. participation in the Vietnam War
    d. witnessing a friend or relative die from a traumatic event

14) Several surveys have found that approximately _____ of U.S. women have been victims of rape.

    a. 10%
    b. 20%
    c. 30%
    d. 40%

15) This uses laboratory equipment to monitor physiological processes that generally occur outside of conscious awareness to help individuals learn how to control their autonomic nervous system functions voluntarily.

    a. biofeedback
    b. stress management
    c. systematic desensitization
    d. flooding

16) _____ is the most important goal of intervention with cardiovascular disease.

    a. Medication
    b. Prevention
    c. Psychotherapy
    d. Education

17) According to the Social Re-Adjustment Rating Scale, _____ is the most significant life event that constitutes the greatest number of life change units.

    a. pregnancy
    b. divorce
    c. foreclosure of a mortgage or loan
    d. death of one's spouse

18) Psychoneuroimmunology refers to:

    a. the study of decreased production of T cells and other immune agents
    b. the study of inhibition and destruction of various immune agents

c. the study of the effects of stress on the functioning of the immune system

d. the study of white blood cells that fight off foreign substances that invade the body

19) All of the following are factors that increase the risk for experiencing trauma and therefore make PTSD more likely EXCEPT:

a. having a history of conduct problems during childhood

b. being male

c. being less educated

d. having an introverted personality

20) (A) _____ amount of stress is healthy for the heart.

a. small

b. moderate

c. large

d. No

21) Psychologists in this field define disease as "dis-ease", indicating that illness is a departure not only from adaptive biological functioning but also from adaptive social and psychological functioning.

a. biopsychosocial psychology

b. behavioral psychology

c. health psychology

d. dynamic psychology

22) As many as _____ of all stranger rapes are not reported to authorities.

a. one-third

b. two-thirds

c. one-quarter

d. one-half

23) According to the Framingham Study which was reviewed in your textbook, which of the following is most likely to suffer from heart disease?

a. a woman who is a homemaker and has two children

b. a woman who is a homemaker and has four children

c. a woman who is a sales manager and has two children

d. a woman who is a waitress and has four children

24) Some research indicates that it is helpful to recount stressful experiences because:

   a. it can reduce the various psychophysiological indicators of the
      stress response
   b. it helps dissipate negative feelings associated with the stressful
      experiences
   c. it helps the individual to "let go" of the experience and continue on
      with his or her life
   d. there is no research that supports the effectiveness of recounting
      stressful experiences

25) Studies have found that _____ is the most effective treatment for people suffering from PTSD.

   a. hypnotherapy
   b. psychodynamic therapy
   c. trauma desensitization
   d. there were no significant differences detected between any of the above therapies

26) _____ is the help and understanding received from friends and family as well as from professionals.

   a. A personal network
   b. Social support
   c. Psychotherapy
   d. none of the above

27) Which of the following is NOT typically a symptom of PTSD:

   a. difficulty falling or staying asleep
   b. irritability or outbursts of anger
   c. paranoid thoughts or ideas
   d. difficulty concentrating

28) This term indicates that a given physical disease is a product of both the mind and the body.

   a. somatoform
   b. cognitive error
   c. dissociative
   d. psychosomatic

29) All of the following are examples of cognitive responses to stress EXCEPT:

    a. control
    b. repression
    c. appraisal
    d. predictability

30) A horrifying experience that leads to general increases in anxiety and arousal, avoidance of emotionally charged situations, and the frequent reliving of the traumatic event is called:

    a. posttraumatic stress disorder (PTSD)
    b. victimization
    c. acute stress disorder
    d. generalized anxiety disorder

BRIEF ESSAY

As a final exercise, write out answers to the following brief essay questions. Then compare your answers with the material presented in the text.

After you have answered these questions, review the "Critical Thinking" questions that are presented at the end of the text chapter. Answering these questions will help you integrate important issues and themes that have been featured throughout the chapter.

1. Discuss Holmes and Rahe's Social Re-Adjustment Rating Scale. How do they define a *life change unit*? What could be considered some of the strengths of this scale? What are some of the criticisms of this scale? How would you change this scale to address some of these criticisms?

2. Briefly discuss Hans Selye's and Walter Cannon's approaches to studying stress. In what ways are they similar? In what ways do they differ?

3. Briefly describe Posttraumatic Stress Disorder (PTSD). Give an example of an experience that may result in PTSD and identify the various symptoms that might accompany this disorder.

4. What does the chapter mean when it states that cardiovascular disease (CVD) is a *lifestyle disease*? What are the implications of this? How has health psychology attempted to address this?

ANSWER KEY

MATCHING EXERCISES

1. r	11. c
2. a	12. q
3. f	13. n
4. s	14. d
5. l	15. h
6. o	16. b
7. m	17. g
8. t	18. e
9. i	19. k
10. p	20. j

MULTIPLE CHOICE EXERCISES

1.	d	6.	b	11. c	
2.	d	7.	d	12. a	
3.	c	8.	c	13. c	
4.	a	9.	d	14. b	
5.	d	10.	b	15. a	

16.	b	21.	c	26. b	
17.	d	22.	b	27. c	
18.	c	23.	d	28. d	
19.	d	24.	a	29. b	
20.	b	25.	d	30. a	

CHAPTER EIGHT
DISSOCIATIVE AND SOMATOFORM DISORDERS

CHAPTER OUTLINE

Introduction
        Brief Historical Perspective: Hysteria and Unconscious Processes
                Unconscious Processes and Contemporary Cognitive Science
                Hysteria and Contemporary Diagnosis

Dissociative Disorders
        Typical Symptoms and Associated Features
        Classification
        The Three Faces of Eve: The Case of Chris Sizemore
        Epidemiology
                Disorder or Role Enactment
        Etiological Considerations and Research
                Biological Factors
                Psychological Factors
                Social Factors
        Treatment of Dissociative Disorders

Somatoform Disorders
        Typical Symptoms and Associated Features
        Unnecessary Medical Treatment
        Classification
                Body Dysmorphic Disorder
                Hypochondriasis
                Somatization Disorder
                Pain Disorder
                Conversion Disorder
        Epidemiology
                Comorbidity
        Etiological Considerations and Research
                Biological Factors
                        Diagnosis by Exclusion
                        Psychological Factors
                              Primary and Secondary Gain
                        Social Factors
        Treatment of Somatoform Disorders

LEARNING OBJECTIVES

After reviewing the material presented in this chapter, you should be able to:

* distinguish dissociative and somatoform disorders

* describe the views on hysteria of: early Greeks, Charcot, Janet, and Freud and compare these perspectives with the contemporary perspective

* define dissociation and psychogenic amnesia

* explain the connection between psychological trauma and fugue, amnesia, and multiple personality disorder

* define retrograde, posttraumatic, anterograde, and selective amnesia

* identify the DSM criteria for depersonalization disorder and multiple personality disorder

* define prosopagnosia and explain the significance of this biologically based disorder for the biological approach to dissociation

* understand the psychological view of dissociative disorders, but be aware that little scientific research has been conducted to verify these theories

* describe the ways in which hypnosis and abreaction presumably aid in the integration of dissociated memories

* give the DSM-IV criteria for body dysmorphic disorder, hypochondriasis, somatization disorder, pain disorder, and conversion disorder

* understand the way in which misdiagnosis of somatoform disorder can be dangerous

* explain Freud's theory of primary and secondary gain used to describe somatoform symptoms

* describe the behavioral therapy approach to treatment of chronic pain

* outline the way physicians should treat the patient who presents "excessive" physical concerns which are not physiologically based

KEY TERMS AND CONCEPTS

Following is a list of key terms and concepts that are featured in the chapter and are important for you to know. Write out the definitions of each of these terms and check your answers with the definitions in the text.

Dissociative disorders
Malingering
Somatoform disorders
Dissociative fugue
Hysteria
Dissociation
Déjà vu experience
Hidden observer
Psychogenic amnesia
Retrograde amnesia
Posttraumatic amnesia
Anterograde amnesia
Selective amnesia
Hypnosis
Depersonalization disorder
Dissociative identity disorder
Multiple personality disorder
Prosopagnosia
Retrospective reports
Recovered memories
State-dependent learning
Iatrogenesis
Abreaction
Body dysmorphic disorder
Hypochondriasis
Somatization disorder
Pseudoneurologic symptoms
La belle indifference
Briquet's syndrome
Pain disorder
Conversion disorder
Diagnosis by exclusion
Primary gain
Secondary gain
Retrospective reports

KEY NAMES

The following individuals have made important contributions to the material presented in the chapter. Write out the names of these individuals and the theories, research, or treatment with which they are associated. Then check your answers with the information in your text.

Jean Charcot
Pierre Janet
Sigmund Freud
Nicholas Spanos

MATCHING QUESTIONS

Match the following terms and names with the definitions presented below. The answers can be found at the end of the chapter.

a. malingering
b. abreaction
c. psuedoneurologic symptom
d. Pierre Janet
e. déjà vu experience
f. Briquet's syndrome
g. prosopagnosia
h. Nicholas Spanos
i. la belle indifference
j. selective amnesia

k. retrospective report
l. somatoform disorders
m. Jean Charcot
n. hysteria
o. recovered memories
p. dissociative disorders
q. retrograde amnesia
r. dissociative identity disorder
s. depersonalization
t. secondary gain

1) ____ loss of memory for events before a particular trauma

2) ____ the strange and brief feeling that an event has happened before

3) ____ the emotional reliving of a traumatic experience

4) ____ a type of dissociative experience wherein people feel detached from their bodies or parts of their bodies

5) ____ pretending to have a disorder in order to achieve some gain

6) ____ evaluations of the past from the vantage point of the present

7) ____ the first person to use hypnosis to treat and induce hysteria

8) _____ a flippant lack of concern about physical symptoms displayed by an individual

9) _____ a group of disorders characterized by disruptions in the integration of memory, consciousness, or identity

10) _____ French philosophy professor who conducted experiments on dissociation, viewing dissociation as an abnormal process

11) _____ another name for somatization disorder

12) _____ physical complaints that mimic neurological diseases

13) _____ a type of impairment of face recognition

14) _____ a process whereby symptoms serve to avoid responsibility and gain attention and sympathy

15) _____ recollections of forgotten traumatic memories

16) _____ a group of disorders characterized by unusual physical symptoms occuring in the absence of a known physical illness

17) _____ loss of memory for selected personal events and information

18) _____ an influential Canadian psychologist who proposed that multiple personalities are caused by role-playing

19) _____ a disorder described in ancient Greece, the term originally meaning "wandering uterus"

20) _____ a condition also known as multiple personality disorder, characterized by the existence of two or more personalities in one person

MULTIPLE CHOICE QUESTIONS

The following multiple choice questions will test your comprehension of the material presented in the chapter. Circle the correct choice for each question in the section. Then compare your answers with those at the end of the chapter.

1) Sudden, unplanned travel, the inability to remember certain past details, and confusion about one's identity are primary features of:

   a. general amnesia
   b. Briquet's syndrome
   c. body dysmorphic disorder
   d. dissociative fugue

2) Abnormal fears of having a serious medical disorder, even after a thorough medical evaluation reveals nothing wrong, is characteristic of:

   a. hypochondriasis
   b. depersonalization disorder
   c. somatization disorder
   d. conversion disorder

3) An unfortunate consequence of having a somatoform disorder is:

   a. the patient does not attend to the medical aspects of the disorder, resulting in underutilization of health care
   b. the psychological nature of the patient's problems go unnoticed, and unnecessary medical procedures are performed
   c. the seriousness of the physical complaints are overlooked, and necessary medical treatments are refused
   d. mental health professionals are consulted instead of physicians, resulting in poor physical health care

4) Which disorder does NOT appear to overlap with somatoform disorders?

   a. anxiety disorders
   b. depression
   c. antisocial personality disorder
   d. multiple personality disorder

5) Freud believed that both dissociative and somatoform disorders were:

   a. expressions of unresolved anger
   b. reactions of the superego toward repressed impulses
   c. expressions of unconscious conflict
   d. conscious reactions to traumatic situations

6) "La belle indifference" is occasionally exhibited by patients with:

    a. multiple personality disorder
    b. pain disorder
    c. psychogenic amnesia
    d. somatization disorder

7) Whenever Tom looks into the mirror, the first thing he notices is his large and somewhat pointed ears. Although friends have reassured him otherwise, he is convinced that his ears are the first thing others notice about him, too. In fact, he wonders whether some people may call him Mr. Spock behind his back. He has consulted with several plastic surgeons and his first surgery has just been scheduled. Tom displays symptoms of:

    a. somatization disorder
    b. Briquet's syndrome
    c. conversion disorder
    d. body dysmorphic disorder

8) Sally feels depressed about her relationship with her boyfriend as she studies for her spring chemistry final. The next fall, she enrolls in another chemistry course and finds herself easily remembering the material from her spring course as she studies for her first review quiz. On this occasion, she is also depressed, this time due to a fight with her girlfriend. This could be an example of:

    a. state-dependent learning
    b. abreaction
    c. hypnotic recall
    d. recovered memory

9) How may antianxiety, antipsychotic, or antidepressant medications be helpful in the treatment of dissociative disorders?

    a. they facilitate reintegration of the dissociated states
    b. they reduce the level of the patient's emotional distress
    c. they increase the likelihood of having one personality become dominant
       over other personalities
    d. they are not recommended treatment for dissociative disorders

10) A critical consideration in the diagnosis of a somatoform disorder is:

    a. the person may be aware of the psychological factors producing the
       disorder
    b. the person may minimize his or her physical complaints, resulting in not
       detecting the disorder

c. the person may also have coexisting multiple personalities

d. the person may actually have a real but as yet undetected physical illness

11) Which disorder is NOT a type of somatoform disorder?

a. depersonalization disorder
b. body dysmorphic disorder
c. conversion disorder
d. pain disorder

12) A distinguishing feature of somatization disorder is:

a. the physical complaints involve multiple somatic systems (e.g., gastrointestinal, cardiovascular, reproductive)
b. the physical complaints are limited to only one somatic system
c. the patient appears very serious, obsessive, and emotionally withdrawn
d. the onset of the disorder rarely occurs before age 30

13) The separation of mental processes such as memory or consciousness that are usually integrated is referred to as:

a. abreaction
b. dissocation
c. repression
d. déjà vu

14) Which of the following is the best definition of a conversion symptom?

a. a physical symptom in one part of the body that is actually referred pain or trauma from another part of the body
b. a symptom produced by psychological conflict that mimics a symptom found in a neurological disease
c. a symptom produced by injury which is exacerbated by psychological conflict
d. an emotional symptom such as depressed mood produced by physical trauma

15) When is the diagnosis of a dissociative disorder NOT appropriate?

a. when the patient has a history of child sexual abuse
b. when the dissociative process is abrupt in onset
c. when the patient additionally reports feeling depressed
d. when the dissociation occurs in the presence of substance abuse or organic pathology

16) Joe reports to his family doctor that he has not been able to work for six months because of pain in his legs. A housepainter, he is not able to stand the pain during his work. In fact, lately he can barely walk to the kitchen from his bedroom because of the pain. He did not experience any kind of injury that would explain his present situation. His wife has been taking care of him but is very concerned about the financial strain this is causing. His doctor orders a thorough examination. If the results come back negative, what diagnosis should his doctor consider?

    a. conversion disorder
    b. hypochondriasis
    c. pain disoder
    d. somatoform disorder

17) The onset of a dissociative episode:

    a. is typically abrupt and precipitated by a traumatic event
    b. is slow and insidious in nature
    c. can be traced to certain metabolic deficiencies
    d. typically happens following a severe head injury

18) A conversion symptom that serves the function of protecting the conscious mind by expressing the conflict unconsciously is referred to as:

    a. la belle indifference
    b. primary gain
    c. diagnosis by exclusion
    d. introjection

19) While both disorders involve memory loss, a major difference between dissociative amnesia and dissociative fugue is that:

    a. dissociative fugue is characterized by sudden and unexpected travel away from home
    b. the memory loss in dissociative amnesia has a physical basis
    c. dissociative amnesia is characterized by the emergence of at least one additional personality
    d. dissociative fugue additionally includes persistent feelings of being detached from oneself

20) Research on the prevalence of somatoform disorders suggests:

    a. these disorders appear to be more common than depression in the general population

b. these disorders appear to be less common during war time

c. these disorders appear to be rare in the general population

d. the prevalence of these disorders has increased since Freud's time

21) The sociocultural view of the etiology of somatoform disorders suggests that:

    a. people with education and financial security have greater access to physicians who will listen to their somatic complaints

    b. people in nonindustrialized societies have a greater sense of community and are more likely to describe their inner distress to others in their social network

    c. people in industrialized societies have more opportunity to develop a more sophisticated vocabulary for their physical symptoms

    d. people with less education or financial security have less opportunity to learn how to describe their inner turmoil in psychological terms

22) Who would be at risk for developing a dissociative disorder?

    a. a person with a family history of depression

    b. a person with a history of child sexual abuse

    c. a person with a history of violent behavior

    d. all of the above

23) Why are people with somatoform disorders likely to reject a referral to a mental health professional from their physicians?

    a. people may have difficulty accepting the possibility of the psychological basis to their physical symptoms

    b. people may feel that their physician is belittling their problems

    c. people may feel that their physician is not being empathic

    d. all of the above

24) Which statement is NOT correct about somatization disorder:

    a. it is more common among higher socioeconomic groups

    b. it is more common among women

    c. it is more common among African Americans than Americans of European heritage

    d. somatic symptoms are more frequent among people who have lost a spouse

25) Every Friday Sarah's fifth grade class has a spelling test. Every Friday morning, Sarah complains of a stomachache to her mother. This may be an example of:

    a. expressing an emotional concern that has a genuine emotional basis

    b. expressing an emotional concern in terms of a physical complaint

c. expressing a physical complaint that has been reinforced by the environment

d. expressing a psychological symptom that has an organic basis

26) Somatoform disorders are characterized by:

a. physical complaints that can be traced to organic impairment

b. patients who deliberately lie about the presence of physical symptoms

c. physical symptoms that cannot be explained on the basis of underlying physical illness

d. physical symptoms which are consciously linked to psychological difficulties

27) Although their presenting symptoms differ greatly in appearance, a common link between dissociative and somatoform disorders is:

a. both involve memory loss

b. both require extensive medical treatment

c. both apparently involve unconscious processes

d. all of the above

28) In contrast to Freud, contemporary cognitive scientists:

a. do not recognize the existence of unconscious processes

b. believe that unconscious processes are much less influential in shaping both normal and abnormal behavior

c. believe that unconscious processes are more influential than conscious processes in shaping both normal and abnormal behavior

d. have a much less restricted view of unconscious processes and their role in shaping behavior

29) The analogue experiments conducted by Spanos and his colleagues on the symptoms of multiple personality disorder suggest that:

a. hypnosis had no relationship to the presence of symptoms of this disorder

b. the symptoms of this disorder disappeared under hypnosis

c. the symptoms of this disorder can be induced through role-playing and hypnosis

d. experimental hypnosis increases risk for the onset of multiple personality disorder

30) An example of a sociological theory of the etiology of multiple personality disorder (MPD) is:
   - a. MPD is caused by disturbances in the temporal lobe of the brain
   - b. MPD is caused by a perceptual disturbance that impairs the ability to recognize faces
   - c. MPD is produced by iatrogenesis, specifically, through the leading questions of therapists
   - d. MPD is produced by recovered memories of the loss of a parent

BRIEF ESSAY

As a final exercise, write out answers to the following brief essay questions. Then compare your answers with the material presented in the text.

After you have answered these questions, review the "Critical Thinking" questions that are presented at the end of the text chapter. Answering these questions will help you integrate important issues and themes that have been featured throughout the chapter.

1. While some professionals believe that multiple personalities are real and more common than previously thought, others believe that the condition is no more than role-playing. Discuss this controversy, citing the research and clinical evidence that supports both points of view.

2. Are recovered memories examples of dissociation or are they produced through the power of suggestion? Defend your own position on this controversial topic.

3. Review the methodological concerns surrounding the use of retrospective reports. What are the important questions that have been raised regarding their reliability and validity? What are the implications of these concerns regarding the use of retrospective reports in research?

4. Pretend that you are a primary care physician with a patient who has presented with a number of vague and inconsistent physical complaints. An extensive medical evaluation reveals no organic pathology. Discuss the types of questions you would ask yourself in trying to determine whether the patient has a somatoform disorder. What would be your approach to the treatment of this patient if a diagnosis of somatization disorder was given?

ANSWER KEY

MATCHING EXERCISES

1. q	11. f
2. e	12. c
3. b	13. g
4. s	14. t
5. a	15. o
6. k	16. l
7. m	17. j
8. i	18. h
9. p	19. m
10. d	20. r

MULTIPLE CHOICE EXERCISES

1. d	6. d	11. a
2. a	7. d	12. a
3. b	8. a	13. b
4. d	9. b	14. b
5. c	10. d	15. d

16. c	21. d	26. c
17. a	22. b	27. c
18. b	23. d	28. b
19. a	24. a	29. c
20. c	25. b	30. c

CHAPTER NINE
PERSONALITY DISORDERS

CHAPTER OUTLINE

Overview

Typical Symptoms and Associated Features
    Temperament
    Personality

Classification
    Axis II: Specific Subtypes in DSM-IV
        Cluster A
        Cluster B
        Cluster C
    A Dimensional Perspective on Classification

Epidemiology
    Prevalence Among Adults in Community Samples
    Prevalence Among Patients
    Stability Over Time
    Gender Bias

Schizotypal Personality Disorder (SPD)
    Brief Historical Perspective
    Clinical Features and Co-morbidity
    Etiological Considerations
    Treatment

Borderline Personality Disorder (BPD)
    Brief Historical Perspective
    Clinical Features and Co-morbidity
    Etiological Considerations
    Treatment

Antisocial Personality Disorder (APD)
    Brief Historical Perspective
    Clinical Features and Co-morbidity

Etiological Considerations
  Genetic Factors
  Family Factors
  Avoidance Learning and Disinhibition
  Treatment

Summary

LEARNING OBJECTIVES

After reviewing the material presented in this chapter, you should be able to:

*   appreciate the fact that the person who has a personality disorder's behavior is ego-syntonic

*   define temperament and the broader term, personality and explain the relevance of these concepts to the study of personality disorders

*   classify the personality disorders into the three clusters according to the categories: eccentric, dramatic, and anxious

*   provide a basic description of each of the ten DSM-IV personality disorders

*   compare and contrast the avoidant personality disorder and the dependent personality disorder

*   know the basic prevalence rates for personality disorders in general and which are the most and least common specific personality disorders

*   describe the key clinical features of schizotypal personality disorder, borderline personality disorder, and antisocial personality disorder

*   compare the treatments of schizotypal, borderline, and antisocial personality disorder patients

KEY TERMS AND CONCEPTS

Following is a list of key terms and concepts that are featured in the chapter and are important for you to know. Write out the definitions of each of these terms and check your answers with the definitions in the text.

Personality
Personality disorder

Antisocial personality disorder
Ego-dystonic
Ego-syntonic
Narcissistic personality disorder
Histrionic personality disorder
Temperament
Person-situation debate
Interactional
General response style
Aggregated assessments
Neuroticism
Extraversion
Openness to experience
Agreeableness
Conscientiousness
Paranoid personality disorder
Schizoid personality disorder
Schizotypal personality disorder
Borderline personality disorder
Avoidant personality disorder
Dependent personality disorder
Obsessive-compulsive personality disorder
Schedule for Nonadaptive and Adaptive Personality (SNAP)
Schizophrenia
Schizoid
Simple schizophrenia
Smooth-pursuit eye movements (SPEM)
Primary process thinking
Splitting
Primate separation model
Dialectical behavior therapy
Moral insanity
Psychopathic insanity
Psychopath
Adoptees
Criminal behavior
Adolescence-limited antisocial behavior
Life-course-persistent antisocial behavior

KEY NAMES

The following individuals have made important contributions to the material presented in
the chapter. Write out the names of these individuals and the theories, research, or

treatment with which they are associated. Then check your answers with the information in your text.

Hervey Cleckley
Arnold Buss
Robert Plomin
Michael Rutter
Thomas Widiger
David Bernstein
Patricia Cohen
Larry Siever
Otto Kernberg
John Gunderson
Hagop Akiskal
Lee Robins
Terrie Moffitt

MATCHING QUESTIONS

Match the following terms and names with the definitions presented below. The answers can be found at the end of the chapter.

a. moral insanity
b. simple schizophrenia
c. ego-syntonic
d. dialectical behavior therapy
e. Lee Robins
f. primate separation model
g. primary process thinking
h. interactional view of personality
i. psychopathy
j. life-course-persistent antisocial behavior

k. temperament
l. aggregated assessments
m. Otto Kernberg
n. personality
o. ego-dystonic
p. splitting
q. extroversion
r. Hervey Cleckley
s. neuroticism
t. adolescent-limited antisocial behavior

1) _____ symptomatic thoughts, feelings, and behaviors are experienced as foreign or outside of the personality, causing the person distress

2) _____ a common form of often adaptive social behavior that disappears by the time the person becomes an adult

3) _____ a historical term referring to persons who are not psychotic but display symptoms similar to those of schizophrenia

4) _____ a psychiatrist who has developed a psychodynamic theory-based

111

explanation for the development of borderline personality disorder

5) _____   a promising treatment for borderline individuals that combines behavioral techniques with the principles of supportive psychotherapy

6) _____   a term describing individuals who are impulsive, self-centered, and pleasure-seeking, and who do not appear to experience anxiety or guilt about their behavior

7) _____   a type of thought process characterized by a lack of impulse control and in which the id relieves tensions by imagining the things it desires

8) _____   symptomatic thoughts, feelings, and behaviors are experienced as part of the person's self and are viewed as acceptable

9) _____   a prominent researcher who demonstrated that certain types of conduct problems in childhood can reliably predict other forms of adult antisocial behavior

10) _____   refers to individual differences in numerous behavioral tendencies, particularly those which manifest themselves during the first year of life

11) _____   the tendency to see persons and events alternately as entirely good or entirely bad

12) _____   a theoretical factor of personality that refers to activity level, particularly the person's level of ease and comfort in social situations and expressing positive emotions

13) _____   a historical term referring to persistent patterns of immoral and criminal behavior

14) _____   proposed as an explanation for the development of mood disorders, this is a theory of social development in monkeys based on observations of infant monkeys who have been separated from their mothers

15) _____   a broad term referring to patterns of behavior that a person develops in response to coping with both innate traits and abilities and the person's social environment

16) _____   antisocial behavior manifested in a variety of ways, which begins in childhood and continues throughout the person's life

17) ____ a psychiatrist whose clinical descriptions of and ideas about antisocial individuals have been extremely influential in shaping current views on antisocial personality disorder

18) ____ a method of measurement that involves acquiring a composite rating of a behavior based on several observations over time

19) ____ a view of personality that proposes that behavior is the product of both situations and personality traits

20) ____ a theoretical factor of personality that is concerned with the expression of emotional stability

MULTIPLE CHOICE QUESTIONS

The following multiple choice questions will test your comprehension of the material presented in the chapter. Circle the correct choice for each question in the section. Then compare your answers with those at the end of the chapter.

1) John is always on the lookout for potential harm. He has difficulty trusting anyone, even family members, and is consistently suspicious of their motives. He is oversensitive to minor events, reading into them ulterior meanings. His manner of relating to people has caused him problems at work and home. A good diagnosis for John would be:

    a. schizoid personality disorder
    b. obsessive-compulsive personality disorder
    c. antisocial personality disorder
    d. paranoid personality disorder

2) The overall lifetime prevalence of personality disorders in the general population is approximately:

    a. 5 - 9%
    b. 10 - 14%
    c. 15 - 19%
    d. 20 - 24%

3) Which of the following is a criterion which is used in DSM-IV to define personality disorders?

    a. the person must be aware of how his or her behavior is maladaptive
    b. the person's behavior must be rigid and inflexible
    c. the person's behavior must cause legal problems
    d. the person's behavioral difficulties must have started in childhood

4) Which of the following statements represents an approach that has been used to conceptualize personality disorders?

    a. personality disorders are types of personality styles that are closely associated with specific forms of adult psychopathology
    b. personality disorders result from problems in childhood development as conceptualized by psychodynamic theories
    c. personality disorders are manifestations of the presence of specific psychological deficits
    d. all of the above

5) The most common Axis I disorder co-diagnosed with borderline personality disorder is:

    a. depression
    b. substance abuse
    c. anxiety
    d. sexual dysfunction

6) In her longitudinal research on antisocial behavior, Robins found that which of the following was associated with an increased probability of antisocial personality in adulthood?

    a. a sibling with a diagnosis of antisocial personality
    b. a history of substance abuse in the child's mother
    c. inconsistent discipline or absence of discipline in the family
    d. neurological abnormalities in childhood

7) One of the most important characteristics of personality disorders as defined by DSM-IV is:

    a. they are typically experienced as ego-syntonic
    b. the impairment associated with these disorders is more severe than is found in other forms of mental disorder
    c. they are episodic and time-limited in nature
    d. they are consistently reliably diagnosed

8) Research focusing on relationships among personality disorders suggests that:

    a. there is little diagnostic overlap across all personality disorder categories
    b. histrionic personality disorder demonstrates the least amount of diagnostic overlap with other personality disorder categories
    c. there is considerable overlap across diagnostic categories
    d. obsessive-compulsive personality disorder demonstrates the greatest

amount of overlap with other personality disorders

9) The most common personality disorder in both inpatient and outpatient settings is probably:

a. dependent personality disorder
b. antisocial personality disorder
c. borderline personality disorder
d. paranoid personality disorder

10) Which statement is correct regarding treatment of personality disorders?

a. people with personality disorders benefit most from insight-oriented psychotherapy
b. people with personality disorders who present for treatment often do so because they have another type of mental disorder such as depression
c. people with personality disorders benefit most from antipsychotic drugs
d. people with personality disorders who present for treatment usually remain in treatment until it is completed

11) The most common axis I disorder present in individuals with a diagnosis of antisocial personality disorder is:

a. dissociative fugue
b. depression
c. schizophrenia
d. substance abuse

12) Which of the following is considered the primary feature of borderline personality disorder?

a. consistent instability in self-image, mood, and interpersonal relationships
b. extreme social anxiety
c. consistent disregard for authority figures
d. extreme fear of rejection from others

13) Approximately _____ of people with personality disorders do NOT seek professional treatment.

a. 40%
b. 60%
c. 80%
d. 95%

14) Tom is definitely a loner. He has no close friends and appears to be indifferent to relationships. Other people would describe Tom as distant and aloof. In addition, Tom reports that he does not feel strongly about anything. He can't think of anything that really makes him excited; then again, he doesn't get upset or distressed about anything either. Tom might qualify for which of the following personality disorders?

    a. borderline
    b. schizoid
    c. paranoid
    d. narcissistic

15) Which of the following is NOT a primary temperamental trait manifested in early life as suggested by the work of Buss and Plomin?

    a. emotionality
    b. impulsivity
    c. activity
    d. conscientiousness

16) Which of the following has NOT been a proposed explanation for the etiology of borderline personality disorder?

    a. early substance abuse
    b. negative consequences resulting from parental loss during childhood
    c. a history of physical and sexual abuse
    d. problematic relationships with parents

17) Personality disorders are listed on which axis of DSM-IV?

    a. I
    b. II
    c. III
    d. IV

18) Which statement regarding gender differences in personality disorders is correct?

    a. antisocial personality disorder appears to be more frequently diagnosed
       in women
    b. men seek treatment for their personality disorders more often than women
    c. the overall prevalence of personality disorders is approximately equal
       in men and women
    d. histrionic personality disorder is more likely to be diagnosed in men

19) Which of the following would NOT be considered a characteristic feature of antisocial personality disorder?

    a. emotional instability
    b. failure to conform to social norms
    c. deceitfulness
    d. irritability and aggressiveness

20) Mary reports that she feels lonely and isolated. Although she has good relationships with family members, she is so afraid of negative criticism from others that she tends to distance herself from relationships. She desparately wants to make friends, but is afraid of being rejected. She constantly watches for even minimal signs of disapproval. Which personality disorder diagnosis is most appropriate for Mary?

    a. schizoid
    b. histrionic
    c. narcisstic
    d. avoidant

21) An advantage of a dimensional system of classifying personality disorders would be:

    a. it would eliminate the need for diagnosis
    b. personality disorders would be more reliably assessed
    c. it would be more useful for those individuals whose symptoms and
       behaviors fall on the boundaries between different personality disorder
       diagnoses
    d. it would require less time to arrive at a diagnosis

22) Studies investigating the long-term course of antisocial personality disorder indicate that:

    a. antisocial individuals tend to become more careless as they grow older,
       resulting in increasing numbers of arrests
    b. antisocial individuals continue their criminal activity well into middle age
    c. antisocial individuals tend to reform their behavior after several incarcerations
    d. people exhibiting antisocial behavior tend to 'burn out' when they reach middle
       age

23) According to the five-factor model of personality, the willingness to cooperate and empathize with other people is the trait referred to as:

    a. conscientiousness
    b. affiliation
    c. agreeableness

d. cooperativeness

24) Larry has extreme difficulty making decisions on his own. He tends to cling to other people and continually asks them for assistance in making even minor decisions. In addition, he constantly asks for his friends' advice and wants to be reassured about everything, even his ability to be a friend. A possible diagnosis for Larry might be:

a. dependent personality disorder
b. avoidant personality disorder
c. narcissistic personality disorder
d. borderline personality disorder

25) Individual psychotherapy with borderline patients can be difficult because:

a. borderline patients frequently cannot afford the cost of such treatment
b. borderline patients are often so transient that it is difficult for them to remain in treatment for more than a brief period of time
c. maintaining the type of concentration necessary for individual therapy is particularly difficult for such patients
d. establishing and maintaining the type of close relationship necessary between therapist and patient is particularly difficult for borderlines

26) Research on the biological correlates of schizotypal personality disorder suggests that:

a. 75% of individuals who meet criteria for schizotypal personality have a first-degree relative with schizophrenia
b. SPEM (eye-tracking) abnormalities in a college-student population are associated with the presence of characteristic features of schizotypal personality disorder
c. SPEM abnormalities are most likely to be present in persons with particular schizotypal characteristics, namely, odd thinking and speech
d. all of the above

27) Research on the genetics of antisocial personality disorder suggests which of the following statements?

a. genetic and environmental factors combine in the production of criminal behavior
b. the presence of any type of genetic factor in the production of antisocial behavior is dubious
c. without the presence of genetic factors, environmental factors alone can never predict the development of criminal behavior
d. environmental factors are much more important than genetic factors in the production of criminal behavior

28) The personality disorders listed in DSM-IV are divided into how many clusters?

    a. 2
    b. 3
    c. 4
    d. 5

29) Sally takes pride in efficient performance and rational behavior. While others see her as rigid, perfectionistic, inflexible, and judgmental, Sally believes that others simply do not share the same standards and are not worthy of her high opinion. She does not show affection and finds 'mushy' feelings in others distasteful. Which personality disorder might Sally have?

    a. schizotypal personality disorder
    b. antisocial personality disorder
    c. obsessive-compulsive personality disorder
    d. schizoid personality disorder

30) Which statement regarding treatment of antisocial personalities is correct?

    a. treatment is usually successful if the individual does not have a
       history of legal difficulties
    b. currently the best treatment available for this disorder is family therapy
    c. approximately two-thirds of individuals with this disorder show clinical
       improvement if treated with psychodynamic therapy
    d. the presence of depression in people with this disorder may be associated with a
       better prognosis for treatment for this disorder

BRIEF ESSAY

As a final exercise, write out answers to the following brief essay questions. Then compare your answers with the material presented in the text.

After you have answered these questions, review the "Critical Thinking" questions that are presented at the end of the text chapter. Answering these questions will help you integrate important issues and themes that have been featured throughout the chapter.

1. Describe the five-factor model of personality. What are the five factors and their definitions? What would be characteristics of low and high scorers on these traits?

2. Discuss the problems associated with the treatment of individuals with personality disorders. Why is a poor prognosis for treatment associated with most of these disorders? What treatment approaches seem most promising to you?

3. Review the controversies that surround the issue of stability of personality. What methods have been used in the attempt to demonstrate stable traits? What do you think are methodological limitations of these approaches?

4. Pretend that you are on the committee to develop DSM-V. Would you recommend classifying personality disorders using a dimensional or categorical approach? Why?

ANSWER KEY

MATCHING EXERCISES

1. o	11. p
2. t	12. q
3. b	13. a
4. m	14. f
5. d	15. n
6. i	16. j
7. g	17. r
8. c	18. l
9. e	19. h
10. k	20. s

MULTIPLE CHOICE EXERCISES

1. d	6. c	11. d
2. b	7. a	12. a
3. b	8. c	13. c
4. d	9. c	14. b
5. a	10. b	15. d

16. a	21. c	26. b
17. b	22. d	27. a
18. c	23. c	28. b
19. a	24. a	29. c
20. d	25. d	30. d

CHAPTER TEN
ALCOHOLISM AND SUBSTANCE USE DISORDERS

CHAPTER OUTLINE

Overview

Typical Symptoms and Associated Features
    Short-term Effects of Alcohol
    Patterns of Consumption
        Craving
        Diminished Control
    Tolerance and Withdrawal
    Consequences of Prolonged Abuse

Classification
    Brief History of Legal and Illegal Substances
        Jellinek's Phases of Alcoholism
        Early Classification Systems
    Contemporary Diagnostic Systems (DSM-IV)
    Proposed Subtypes of Alcoholism
    Course and Outcome
    Other Disorders Commonly Associated with Addictions

Epidemiology
    Incidence, Prevalence, and Morbid Risk
        Other Drugs
    Gender Differences
    Risk for Addiction across the Life Span

Etiological Considerations and Research
    Early Stages: Initiation and Continuation
    Middle Stages: Escalation and Transition to Abuse
        Genetics of Alcoholism
            Twin Studies
            Adoption Studies
        Neurochemical Modes of Action
            Endogenous Opioid Receptors
            The Serotonin Hypothesis
        Psychological Factors
            Expectations about the Effects of Alcohol
            Attention Allocation
    Advanced Stages: Tolerance and Withdrawal

Treatment
> Detoxification and Pharmacotherapy
>> Disulfiram (Antabuse)
> Self-help Groups: Alcoholics Anonymous
> Controlled Drinking
> Relapse Prevention
> General Conclusions Regarding Treatment

Summary

LEARNING OBJECTIVES

After reviewing the material presented in this chapter, you should be able to:

*   distinguish substance abuse and substance dependence

*   define tolerance and withdrawal

*   name some of the main consequences of extended drug or alcohol abuse

*   describe Jelinek's phases of alcoholism

*   identify some of the main gender differences in alcohol use and abuse

*   describe the development of alcoholism according to early, middle, and later stages

*   state some of the basic findings regarding the genetics of alcoholism--from twin and adoption studies

*   explain the endorphin hypothesis and the serotonin hypothesis

*   understand the importance of cognitive expectations in the effects of alcohol

*   describe the following treatment programs: detoxification, self-help groups, controlled drinking training, and relapse prevention training

KEY TERMS AND CONCEPTS

Following is a list of key terms and concepts that are featured in the chapter and are important for you to know. Write out the definitions of each of these terms and check your answers with the definitions in the text.

Substance dependence
Tolerance
Withdrawal
Substance abuse
Polysubstance abuse
Addiction
Psychoactive substance
Hypnotics
Sedatives (anxiolytics)
CNS stimulants
Opiates (narcotic analgesics)
Cannibinoids
Alcohol intoxication
Concealed drinking
Psychological dependence
Delirium
Delirium tremens
Blackouts
Amnestic disorders
Prealcoholic phase
Prodromal phase
Crucial phase
Chronic phase
Endorphins
Neuropeptides
Tension-reduction hypothesis
Balanced placebo design
Attention-allocation model
Drunken excess
Drunken self-inflation
Drunken relief
Inhibition conflict
Anticipatory compensation
Drug compensatory response
Release from tolerance
Compensatory hyperthermic response
Detoxification
Disulfiram (Antabuse)
Controlled drinking
Abstinence violation effect

KEY NAMES

The following individuals have made important contributions to the material presented in the chapter. Write out the names of these individuals and the theories, research, or treatment with which they are associated. Then check your answers with the information in your text.

E. M. Jellinek
Robert Cloninger
George Vaillant
Matt McGue
Donald Goodwin
Michael Bohman
Claude Steele
Robert Josephs
Shephard Siegel
Mark and Linda Sobell
Alan Marlatt

MATCHING QUESTIONS

Match the following terms and names with the definitions presented below. The answers can be found at the end of the chapter.

a. binges
b. alcohol intoxication
c. balanced placebo design
d. opiates
e. Robert Cloninger
f. anticipatory compensation
g. tolerance
h. stimulants
i. cannibinoids
j. delirium tremens

k. E. M. Jellinek
l. hypnotics
m. detoxification
n. concealed drinking
o. withdrawal
p. blackout
q. tension-reduction hypothesis
r. sedatives
s. abstinence violation effect
t. endorphins

1) _____ a type of CNS depressant, a class of drugs that relieve anxiety and are also referred to as anxiolytics

2) _____ the consequent guilt and perceived loss of control that a person experiences whenever he or she takes a drink (relapses) following an extended period of abstinence

3) _____ often occuring in alcohol abusers, this experience is characterized

124

by the inability to remember a specific period of time when the person was under the influence of alcohol

4) _____ neuropeptides which are naturally synthesized in the brain and are closely related to morphine in terms of their pharmacological properties

5) _____ an influential researcher who described alcoholism as a progressive disorder resulting in either abstinence or death

6) _____ symptoms of this clinical state include slurred speech, lack of coordination, unsteady gait, impaired attention or memory, and occasionally stupor and coma

7) _____ a type of CNS depressant, this type of medication helps induce sleep

8) _____ episodes of prolonged and uninterrupted drinking and intoxication

9) _____ a pathological pattern of abuse involving the consumption of alcohol when alone or not being observed

10) _____ nicotine and caffeine are examples of this type of drug

11) _____ the theory that people drink alcohol in order to reduce the impact of a stressful environment

12) _____ also referred to as narcotic analgesics, this class of drugs can be used to decrease pain

13) _____ a psychiatrist who has proposed two different subtypes of alcoholism with genetic factors playing differing roles in each subtype

14) _____ the process through which a person's nervous system becomes less sensitive to the effects of a substance such as alcohol

15) _____ an effect produced by many drugs in which the unconditioned response's (UCR) effect opposes that of the unconditioned stimulus (UCS)

16) _____ the often gradual process of removing a drug on which a person has become dependent

17) _____ a type of drug that can produce a sense of well-being and an altered sense of time

18) _____ a syndrome caused by withdrawal from alcohol that is characterized

125

by disturbance of consciousness and changes in cognitive processing

19) _____ a type of research method which allows the separation of the biological effects of the drug from subject expectations about the effect of the drug on his or her behavior

20) _____ unpleasant psychological and/or physical effects experienced by a person when he or she stops taking a substance after its prolonged use (only certain substances can produce such effects)

MULTIPLE CHOICE QUESTIONS

The following multiple choice questions will test your comprehension of the material presented in the chapter. Circle the correct choice for each question in the section. Then compare your answers with those at the end of the chapter.

1) The two terms included in the DSM-IV to describe substance use disorders are:

    a. substance dependence and substance abuse
    b. substance abuse and addiction
    c. tolerance and addiction
    d. substance abuse and polysubstance abuse

2) Although disulfiram (antabuse) can effectively block the chemical breakdown of alcohol, people resist using this drug because:

    a. it is an extremely expensive drug to administer
    b. the effect of the drug is very short-lived; that is, it reduces alcohol intake for only a few hours after its ingestion
    c. individuals who use this drug have to monitor their dietary intake
    d. use of the drug produces a dramatically adverse physical reaction

3) Because alcoholism is associated with many diverse problems, distinguishing between people who are dependent on alcohol and those who are not is often determined by which of the following?

    a. the presence of legal problems (e.g., driving under the influence)
    b. whether or not the person reports tolerance to alcohol
    c. the number of problems that the person experiences
    d. the presence of medical problems

4) Research on the long term course of alcohol suggests that:

a. the typical individual is able to successfully stop drinking only after hospitalization

b. the typical individual cycles through periods of alcohol consumption, cessation, and relapse

c. the typical individual rarely experiences relapse after making the decision to stop drinking

d. the typical individual spends approximately 10 years in the alcohol consumption period before making the decision to quit

5) Which of the following is an example of a CNS stimulant?

a. alcohol

b. cocaine

c. morphine

d. hashish

6) Which of the following describes the prealcoholic phase of alcoholism as described by E. M. Jellinek?

a. the person drinks socially and occasionally drinks heavily to relieve tension

b. the person drinks in secret and has occasional blackouts

c. the person drinks on a daily basis

d. the person drinks regularly until totally intoxicated

7) Results from adoption studies focusing on the genetic transmission of alcohol indicate that:

a. the familial nature of alcoholism appears to be at least partially determined by genes; that is, having an alcoholic biological parent increases risk for alcoholism

b. if a person does not have a alcoholic biological parent, having an adopted parent with alcohol problems greatly increases risk for alcoholism

c. having the personality trait of "behavioral overcontrol" increases risk for alcoholism

d. only people with at least one alcoholic biological parent are at risk for alcoholism

8) John currently drinks large amounts of alcohol on a daily basis. He plans his day around when alcohol will be available to him. He drives a certain route home from work that passes two liquor stores in order to ensure that liquor will be available each evening. His weekend activities are planned around the availability of alcohol, and he will not attend social functions where alcohol is absent. Which term best describes John's condition?

a. binge drinker

b. concealed drinker

c. psychological dependence

d. prealcoholic drinker

9) In most states, the current legal limit of alcohol concentration for driving is:

    a. 50 mg percent

    b. 100 mg percent

    c. 150 mg percent

    d. 200 mg percent

10) One reason that risk for substance dependence is increased in elderly people is that:

    a. the elderly demonstrate a reduced sensitivity to drug toxicity and
therefore require higher drug dosages

    b. adult children often encourage their elderly parents to use drugs to
control their nerves

    c. the elderly use prescribed psychoactive drugs more frequently than
compared to other age groups

    d. in fact, there is little risk for substance dependence in the elderly
(less than 1% of the population)

11) A principal assumption of alcohlics anonymous (AA) is:

    a. people need to relapse several times before they will learn to take
their alcohol problem seriously

    b. individuals cannot recover on their own

    c. individuals need to remove themselves from the stressful situations that
trigger alcohol use

    d. with enough help, people can develop effective methods of controlled drinking

12) A person who has a compelling need to use a drug and cannot control or regulate his/her drug use is commonly described as:

    a. in withdrawal

    b. a recreational drug user

    c. intoxicated

    d. addicted

13) Which of the following statement is accurate regarding the definition of substance dependence in the DSM-IV?

    a. evidence of tolerance and withdrawal is required

    b. the individual must exhibit several characteristics that describe a pattern of compulsive use

    c. the person must exhibit characteristics of problematic substance use for at least two years

    d. a prior diagnosis of substance abuse is required before the diagnosis of substance dependence may be considered

14) Which would NOT be considered an example of a common alcohol expectancy?

    a. alcohol decreases power and aggression

    b. alcohol enhances social and physical pleasure

    c. alcohol enhances sexual performance

    d. alcohol increases social assertiveness

15) Aerosol spray, glue, and paint thinner are all examples of which class of psychoactive drugs?

    a. CNS depressants

    b. over-the-counter drugs

    c. solvents

    d. hallucinogens

16) What percentage of MEN in the United States develop problems resulting from prolonged alcohol consumption?

    a. 10%

    b. 20%

    c. 30%

    d. 40%

17) A person CANNOT become intoxicated on which of the following drugs?

    a. nicotine and cannabis

    b. caffeine and inhalants

    c. inhalants and cannabis

    d. caffeine and nicotine

18) Which of the following statements is TRUE regarding alcohol expectancies?

    a. negative expectancies appear to be less powerful than positive expectancies in influencing alcohol use

    b. adolescents do not appear to have strong beliefs about alcohol prior to taking their first drink

    c. expectations regarding alcohol do not predict drinking behaviors

    d. portrayal of alcohol in the mass media does not appear to influence individuals' alcohol expectancies

19) Which of the following statements regarding tolerance is TRUE?

    a. individuals can develop tolerance to all psychoactive drugs over time
    b. certain hallucinogens such as LSD may not lead to the development of tolerance
    c. the most substantial tolerance effects are found among cannabis users
    d. heroin and CNS stimulants do not lead to the development of tolerance

20) Which statement is TRUE regarding the use of alcohol in women?

    a. women are more likely to increase their rates of drinking after becoming parents
    b. women are more likely to reduce their consumption of alcohol following divorce
    c. women who are better educated, employed, and earn a higher income are more likely to drink
    d. women are most likely to drink when they are middle-aged

21) The most controversial aspect of Individualized Behavior Therapy for Alcoholics (IBTA) is:

    a. its exclusion of group meetings for alcoholics
    b. its inclusion of problem-solving techniques that enable the drinker to identify situations which may potentially trigger heavy drinking
    c. its assumption that controlled drinking is a plausible goal for alcoholics
    d. its inclusion of aversive therapy techniques in which the use of alcohol is paired with an aversive stimulus

22) Which of the following statements is TRUE regarding the presence of alcohol dependence over a long period of time?

    a. alcohol dependence always results in Korsakoff's psychosis
    b. alcohol dependence follows opiate dependence and cocaine dependence in terms of potential negative health consequences
    c. nutritional disturbances caused by alcohol dependence can be controlled through appropriate medication
    d. alcohol dependence has more negative health consequences than does abuse of any other substance

23) Which of the following symptoms are side effects of alcohol withdrawal?

    a. hand tremors, sweating, and nausea
    b. anxiety and insomnia

c. convulsions and hallucinations

d. all of the above

24) The most promising neurochemical explanation of alcoholism currently focuses on which of the following neurotransmitters?

a. serotonin

b. dopamine

c. epinephrine

d. norepinephrine

25) Considering all the direct and indirect ways that alcohol use contributes to death (e.g., suicides, accidents, medical disorders), alcohol is considered:

a. the first leading cause of death in this country

b. the second leading cause of death in this country

c. the third leading cause of death in this country

d. the fourth leading cause of death in this country

26) Which of the following statements reflects a difference between men and women in their use of alcohol?

a. the average age of onset for alcoholism is higher among men

b. women are less likely to develop hepatic disorders even after drinking heavily for many years

c. women are more likely to report additional symptoms of depression and anxiety, while antisocial personality traits are more likely to be displayed in men

d. men are more likely to drink if their partners drink

27) Which of the following factors is a predictor of long-term successful treatment outcome for alcoholism?

a. the availability of residential alcohol treatment programs in the area

b. the alcoholic's participation in AA

c. the presence of environmental stress

d. the availability of social support

28) Which class of drugs is LEAST associated with severe withdrawal effects?

a. stimulants

b. alcohol

c. sedatives and anxiolytics

d. opiates

29) One reason that it is difficult to gather epidemiological information on substance use is that:

    a. the definition of substance abuse and dependence has been clearly restricted in the past

    b. this type of research is expensive and therefore has not been adequately funded

    c. drug users are often reluctant to accurately report their drug use because of the illegal status of many drugs

    d. all of the above

30) Which of the following is NOT one of the four phases of alcoholism as described by E. M. Jellinek?

    a. prealcoholic phase

    b. intoxicated phase

    c. crucial phase

    d. chronic phase

BRIEF ESSAY

As a final exercise, write out answers to the following brief essay questions. Then compare your answers with the material presented in the text.

After you have answered these questions, review the "Critical Thinking" questions that are presented at the end of the text chapter. Answering these questions will help you integrate important issues and themes that have been featured throughout the chapter.

1. Discuss the three stages of alcoholism defined in your chapter. What are the defining characteristics and important etiological processes occurring at each stage?

2. Explain Robert Cloninger and Michael Bohman's theory of Type I and Type II alcoholism. What do you think are possible weaknesses of their model? What further type of research is necessary to support or disconfirm such a theory?

3. Describe the balanced placebo design. Why is it a useful research design for the study of the effects of alcohol on behavior?

4. Review the attention-allocation model of alcohol as proposed by Claude Steele and Robert Josephs. What are the two general factors on which this model is based? How does the theory predict such behaviors as drunken excess, drunken self-inflation, and drunken relief?

ANSWER KEY

MATCHING EXERCISES

1. r	11. q
2. s	12. d
3. p	13. e
4. t	14. g
5. k	15. f
6. b	16. m
7. l	17. i
8. a	18. j
9. n	19. c
10. h	20. o

MULTIPLE CHOICE EXERCISES

1. a	6. a	11. b
2. d	7. a	12. d
3. c	8. c	13. b
4. b	9. b	14. a
5. b	10. c	15. c
16. a	21. c	26. c
17. d	22. d	27. d
18. a	23. d	28. a
19. b	24. a	29. c
20. c	25. d	30. b

CHAPTER ELEVEN
SEXUAL AND GENDER IDENTITY DISORDERS

CHAPTER OUTLINE

Classification of sexual disorders
      Brief historical perspective
            Influential clinicians and scientists
            The human sexual response cycle
            Early versions of Diagnostic and Statistical Manual (DSM)
      Homosexuality: A case of politics and diagnosis
      Increased emphasis on sexual dysfunction

Sexual Dysfunction
      Specific subtypes in DSM-IV
            Hypoactive sexual desire disorder
            Sexual aversion disorder
            Male erectile disorder
            Female sexual arousal disorder
            Premature ejaculation
            Female orgasmic disorder
            Pain during sex
      Associated features
            Interpersonal factors and social relationships
      Epidemiology
            Gender differences
            Sexual behavior across the life span
      Etiology
            Sexual desire
            Sexual arousal in men
            Sexual arousal in women
            Premature ejaculation
            Inhibited orgasm
      Treatment
            Sensate focus and scheduling
            Education and cognitive restructuring
            Communication training

Paraphilias
      Typical symptoms and associated features
      Specific subtypes in DSM-IV
            Rape and sexual assault
      Epidemiology
      Etiology

Imprinting and fetishes
Courtship disorders
Intimacy deficits
Vandalized lovemaps
Opponent processes and masochism
Treatment
Aversion therapy
Hormones and medication

Gender identity disorders
Typical symptoms and associated features
Epidemiology
Etiology
Treatment
Sex-reassignment surgery

Summary

LEARNING OBJECTIVES

After reviewing the material presented in this chapter, you should be able to:

* understand that much of our thinking about sexual disorders is a result of cultural and religious values

* know the role of Fred, Ellis, Kinsey, and Masters and Johnson in the study of human sexuality

* distinguish hypoactive sexual desire from sexual aversion disorder

* define male erectile disorder, female arousal disorder, premature ejaculation, dyspareunia, and female orgasmic disorder

* know which sexual disorders are the most common

* list some of the biological and psychological causes of hypoactive sexual desire, disorder of sexual arousal, premature ejaculation, and inhibited orgasm

* describe sensate focus as a treatment technique for sexual disorders

* identify the major forms of paraphilias

135

*   describe some of the causes of paraphilias, including faulty lovemaps, imprinting, courtship disorders, and intimacy deficits

*   distinguish disorders of gender identity from disorders of sexual disorder (e.g., transvestic fetishism).

KEY TERMS AND CONCEPTS

Following is a list of key terms and concepts that are featured in the chapter and are important for you to know. Write out the definitions of each of these terms and check your answers with the definitions in the text.

Sexual dysfunctions
Paraphilias
Sexual perversions
Orgasm
Resolution
Refractory period
Hypoactive sexual desire disorder
Sexual aversion disorder
Female sexual arousal disorder
Male erectile disorder
Female orgasmic disorder (inhibited female orgasm)
Male orgasmic disorder
Premature ejaculation
Dyspareunia
Vaginismus
Erectile dysfunction (impotence)
Inhibited sexual arousal
Operational definition
Penile plethysmograph
Vaginal photometer
Construct validity
Mental scripts
Performance anxiety
Anorgasmic
Sensate focus
Scheduling
Cognitive restructuring
Paraphilias
Exhibitionism
Fetishism
Frotteurism

Pedophilia
Sexual masochism
Sexual sadism
Transvestic fetishism
Voyeurism
Rape
Acquaintance rape
Sadistic rapists
Nonsadistic category of rape
Vindictive rapists
Opportunistic rapists
Imprinting process
Lovemap
Aversion therapy
Gender identity
Sex roles
Gender identity disorder
Transsexualism (gender dysphoria)
Secondary sexual characteristics
Transvestic fetishism
Pseudohermaphroditism
Sex-reassignment surgery

KEY NAMES

The following individuals have made important contributions to the material presented in the chapter. Write out the names of these individuals and the theories, research, or treatment with which they are associated. Then check your answers with the information in your text.

Richard von Krafft-Ebing
Sigmund Freud
Havelock Ellis
Alfred Kinsey
William Masters
Virginia Johnson
Robert Spitzer
Helen Singer Kaplan
Ellen Frank
John Gagnon
William Simon
David Barlow
Raymond Knight

Robert Prentky
Glenn Wilson
Kurt Freund
Ray Blanchard
William Marshall
John Money
Robert Stoller

MATCHING QUESTIONS

Match the following terms and names with the definitions presented below. The answers can be found at the end of the chapter.

a. operational definition
b. performance anxiety
c. paraphilias
d. sensate focus
e. dyspareunia
f. hypoactive sexual desire
g. rape
h. frotteurism
i. transvestic fetishism
j. anorgasmic

k. vaginismus
l. lifelong sexual dysfunction
m. vindictive rapists
n. Glenn Wilson
o. lovemap
p. hypothetical construct
q. opportunistic rapists
r. acquired sexual dysfunction
s. sexual arousal
t. Havelock Ellis

1) _____ this refers to persistent genital pain during or after sexual intercourse

2) _____ this individual has often been called the first sexual modernist

3) _____ considered the cornerstone of sex therapy, this involves a series of simple exercises in which the couple spends time learning to touch each other in a quiet, relaxed setting

4) _____ cross-dressing in heterosexual males

5) _____ disorders in which the characteristic feature is sexual arousal by unusual objects and situations

6) _____ rapists who seem intent on violence directed exclusively toward women and whose actions intend to degrade and humiliate the victim

7) _____ a theoretical device referring to a postulated attribute of a person that helps us understand or explain a person's behavior

8) _____ a sexual response phase preceeding orgasm

9) _____ a mental picture that represents an individual's ideal sexual relationship

10) _____ this term indicates that the problem has been present since the person's first sexual activities

11) _____ this basically includes acts involving nonconsensual sexual penetration

12) _____ this individual explained the development of fetishes in terms of biologically prepared learning

13) _____ rapists who are indifferent to the victim's plight and are seeking immediate gratification through impulsive, unplanned actions

14) _____ becoming an increasingly common reason for referral to a sex clinic, this condition involves a lack of sexual desire

15) _____ touching or rubbing against a nonconsenting person

16) _____ involuntary muscular spasm that causes the muscles of the vagina to snap tightly shut, preventing insertion of any object

17) _____ this term is often used to refer to a "fear of failure"

18) _____ this term indicates that a problem has developed only after a period of normal functioning

19) _____ definition of a theoretical construct in terms of a measurement procedure

20) _____ refers to women who experience inhibited orgasm

MULTIPLE CHOICE QUESTIONS

The following multiple choice questions will test your comprehension of the material presented in the chapter. Circle the correct choice for each question in the section. Then compare your answers with those at the end of the chapter.

1) According to Kurt Freund and Ray Blanchard, all of the following factors may increase the probability that a person might experiment with unusual types of sexual stimulation or employ maladaptive sexual behaviors EXCEPT:

    a. ignorance and poor understanding of human sexuality
    b. lack of diverse sexual experiences
    c. lack of self-esteem
    d. lack of confidence and ability in social interactions

2) All of the following types of medication have been used to treat paraphilias EXCEPT:

    a. antipsychotic medications
    b. antidepressants
    c. antianxiety medications
    d. all of the above have been used to treat paraphilias

3) With regard to the context of occurrence, which of the following terms indicates that the sexual dysfunction is not limited only to certain situations or partners:

    a. situational
    b. lifelong
    c. acquired
    d. generalized

4) Recent revisions of the DSM reflect the following important changes in society's attitudes toward sexual behavior EXCEPT:

    a. growing acceptance of women of their own sexuality
    b. tolerance for greater variety in human sexuality
    c. society's complete acceptance of organized groups that represent
       specific forms of sexual orientation and expression
    d. increased recognition that the main purpose of sexual behavior need not
       be reproduction

5) _____ disorders are more common among women while _____ disorders are more common among men.

    a. orgasm; arousal
    b. arousal; orgasm
    c. aversion; desire
    d. desire; aversion

6) Studies show that most women seeking treatment for hypoactive sexual desire report all of the following EXCEPT:

a. negative perceptions of their parents' attitudes regarding sexual behavior
b. a history of physical and sexual abuse
c. negative perceptions of their parents' demonstration of affection
d. feeling less close to their husbands and having fewer romantic feelings

7) This involves the use of nonliving objects for the purpose of sexual arousal.

a. frotteurism
b. pedophilia
c. fetishism
d. sexual masochism

8) All of the following are secondary sexual characteristics for boys EXCEPT:

a. facial hair
b. voice changes
c. increased muscle mass
d. weight gain

9) Sex-reassignment surgery is the process whereby a person's genitals are changed to match their:

a. gender identity
b. sex role
c. sexual identity
d. gender role

10) According to your text, _____ may be the most common neurologically-based cause of impaired erectile responsiveness among men.

a. depression
b. coronary heart disease
c. diabetes
d. cancer

11) All of the following are treatment options for sexual dysfunctions EXCEPT:

a. sensate focus
b. cognitive restructuring
c. communication training
d. aversion therapy

12) _____ of the people who seek treatment for paraphilia disorders are men.

a. 40%
b. 60%
c. 75%
d. 95%

13) This is a process that resembles that of other species whereby associations are built early in life.

    a. modeling
    b. imprinting
    c. latent learning
    d. observational learning

14) _____ and _____ have undoubtedly been the best-known sex therapists and researchers in the United States since the late 1960's.

    a. William Masters; Virginia Johnson
    b. Alfred Kinsey; Havelock Ellis
    c. Sigmund Freud; Richard von Krafft-Ebing
    d. Robert Spitzer; Helen Singer Kaplan

15) The sense of ourselves as being either male or female is known as:

    a. sexual identity
    b. gender dysphoria
    c. gender identity
    d. sex roles

16) Premature ejaculation may be the most frequent form of sexual dysfunction, affecting nearly 1 in every:

    a. 5 adult men
    b. 10 adult men
    c. 15 adult men
    d. 20 adult men

17) The treatment approach used for paraphilias in which the therapist repeatedly presents a stimulus eliciting inappropriate sexual arousal in association with an aversive stimulus is called:
    a. counterconditioning
    b. aversion therapy
    c. flooding
    d. systematic desensitization

18) Men with this problem may report feeling subjectively aroused, but the vascular reflex mechanism fails, and sufficient blood is not pumped to the penis.

    a. sexual aversion disorder
    b. premature ejaculation
    c. male orgasmic disorder
    d. erectile dysfunction

19) In order to meet diagnostic criteria, all categories of sexual dysfunction require all of the following EXCEPT:

    a. the sexual dysfunction is associated with atypical stimuli and the person is preoccupied with, or consumed by, these activities
    b. the disturbance causes marked distress or interpersonal difficulty
    c. the sexual dysfunction is not better accounted for by another Axis I disorder (such as major depression)
    d. the sexual dysfunction is not due to direct physiological effects of a substance or a general medical condition

20) In their research on sexual behavior across the life span, Masters and Johnson indicated that:
    a. younger men have difficulty regaining an erection if it is lost before orgasm, while older men can only maintain erections for a short period of time
    b. older adults are not as interested in, or capable of, performing sexual behaviors as younger adults
    c. differences between younger and older people are mostly a matter of degree
    d. as women get older, the clitoris becomes more responsive

21) The chapter indicates that perhaps as many as _____ of females seeking treatment for hypoactive sexual desire report other forms of sexual dysfunction.

    a. 25%
    b. 40%
    c. 60%
    d. 75%

22) According to your text, sexual desire remains a controversial topic because:

    a. it is so difficult to define
    b. there is very little empirical research on sexual desire
    c. it is a different construct for men than it is for women
    d. all of the above

23) The unresponsiveness of men to further engage in sexual stimulation for a variable period of time after reaching orgasm is called:

    a. sensation of suspension
    b. pulsation
    c. sexual aversion
    d. refractory period

24) Premature ejaculation might be present if a man is unable to delay ejaculation until his partner reaches orgasm at least _____ of the time.

    a. 25%
    b. 50%
    c. 75%
    d. 100%

25) All of the following refer to one's sense of discomfort with one's anatomic sex EXCEPT:
    a. gender identity disorder
    b. transvestic fetishism
    c. gender dysphoria
    d. transsexualism

26) Studies have shown that all of the following are important factors contributing to failure to reach orgasm among anorgasmic women EXCEPT:

    a. failure to engage in effective behaviors during foreplay
    b. negative attitudes toward masturbation
    c. feelings of guilt about sex
    d. failure to communicate effectively with their partner about sexual
       activities involving direct stimulation of the clitoris

27) Research suggests that _____ of men over age 75 report experiencing erectile dysfunction.

    a. 30%
    b. 40%
    c. 50%
    d. 60%

28) This involves the act of observing an unsuspecting person who is naked, in the process of disrobing, or engaging in sexual activity:

    a. sexual sadism

b. voyeurism

c. exhibitionism

d. fetishism

29) Ellen Frank's study titled "Sexual Problems Reported by 100 `Happily Married' Couples" found all of the following EXCEPT:

a. the frequency of "dysfunctions" (sexual problems that involved sexual arousal and orgasm) and the frequency of "dissatisfactions" (problems associated with the emotional tone of the relationship) were both relatively high

b. women were more likely than their husbands to report almost every type of sexual problem with the exception of reaching orgasm too quickly

c. men indicated difficulty getting excited (an erection) more often than women

d. both women and men reported more dissatisfaction resulting from emotional-type sexual problems than from interference with arousal and orgasm

30) Which of the following characterizes an individual who is genetically male, but is unable to produce a hormone that is responsible for shaping the penis and scrotum in the fetus, and is therefore born with external genitalia that are ambiguous in appearance.

a. transsexualism

b. secondary sexual characteristic disorder

c. transvestic fetishism

d. pseudohermaphroditism

BRIEF ESSAY

As a final exercise, write out answers to the following brief essay questions. Then compare your answers with the material presented in the text.

After you have answered these questions, review the "Critical Thinking" questions that are presented at the end of the text chapter. Answering these questions will help you integrate important issues and themes that have been featured throughout the chapter.

1. Compare and contrast the treatment of paraphilias with the treatment of sexual dysfunction. Choose two types of paraphilias and two types of sexual dysfunctions and discuss which type of treatment you believe would be most effective for each of them.

2. Discuss how von Krafft-Ebing, Freud, Ellis, and Kinsey all contributed to the study of sexual behavior. Discuss some of the similarities and the differences of their contributions.

3. Discuss David Barlow's series of studies comparing sexually dysfunctional men with control subjects in laboratory settings. What were his findings? What are some of the possible limitations to these studies? What are the applications of his findings?

4. Compare and contrast the different proposals regarding the etiology of paraphilias as presented in your text. Which proposal(s) do you believe best explains the etiology of paraphilias? Why?

ANSWER KEY

MATCHING EXERCISES

1. e	11. g
2. t	12. n
3. d	13. q
4. i	14. f
5. c	15. h
6. m	16. k
7. p	17. b
8. s	18. r
9. o	19. a
10. l	20. j

MULTIPLE CHOICE EXERCISES

1. b	6. b	11. d
2. a	7. c	12. d
3. d	8. d	13. b
4. c	9. a	14. a
5. a	10. c	15. c

16. a	21. d	26. a
17. b	22. a	27. c
18. d	23. d	28. b
19. a	24. b	29. c
20. c	25. b	30. d

CHAPTER TWELVE
SCHIZOPHRENIC DISORDERS

CHAPTER OUTLINE

Overview

Typical Symptoms and Course
    Hallucinations
    Delusional Beliefs
    Disorganized Speech
    Motor Disturbances
    Affect and Emotional Disturbances
    Social Withdrawal and Avolition

Classification
    Brief Historical Perspective
        DSM-I and DSM-II
    Contemporary Diagnostic Systems
    Subtypes
        DSM-IV Subcategories
            Disorganized Type
            Catatonic Type
            Paranoid Type
            Undifferentiated Type
            Residual Type
        Positive and Negative Syndromes
    Related Disorders
    Course and Outcome

Epidemiology
    Incidence and Prevalence
    Gender Differences in Onset and Course
    Cross-Cultural Comparisons

Etiological Considerations
    Biological Factors
        Genetics
            Family Studies
            Twin Studies
            Adoption Studies
            The Spectrum of Schizophrenic Disorders
            Linkage Studies
            General Conclusions: A Diathesis-Stress Model

LEARNING OBJECTIVES

After reviewing the material presented in this chapter, you should be able to:

*   distinguish between positive and negative symptoms of schizophrenia

*   define and describe hallucinations, delusional beliefs, and disorganized speech

*   provide examples of typical motor disturbances, affective and emotional disturbances, and avolition

*   understand the contributions of Kraepelin, Bleuler, and Schneider in defining schizophrenia

*   distinguish disorganized, catatonic, paranoid, undifferentiated, and residual types of schizophrenia using DSM-IV criteria

*   describe the following related disorders: schizoaffective disorders, delusional disorder, brief psychotic disorders

*   distinguish the prodromal, active, and residual phases of schizophrenia

*   understand the basic epidemiological statistics for incidence and prevalence of the disorder, as well as gender differences in age of onset

*   understand the genetic evidence for schizophrenia, which leads to a diathesis-stress model of etiology

*   describe some of the research which has discovered structural brain abnormalities for schizophrenics

*   explain the dopamine hypothesis and current beliefs about the role of dopamine in schizophrenia

*   identify some social and psychological factors which may contribute to the development and/or maintenance of schizophrenia

*   understand the significance of research that has identified attentional, cognitive, and eye-tracking dysfunctions in schizophrenics and their biological relatives

*   describe the effectiveness of neuroleptic medication and relevant side effects that are involved in such treatments

*   provide a description of family-oriented aftercare programs, social skills training, and institutional programs in which token economy systems may be used

KEY TERMS AND CONCEPTS

Following is a list of key terms and concepts that are featured in the chapter and are important for you to know. Write out the definitions of each of these terms and check your answers with the definitions in the text.

Negative symptoms

Positive symptoms
Hallucinations
Delusions
Disorganized speech
Thought disorder
Incoherent
Loose associations
Derailment
Tangentiality
Perseveration
Alogia
Poverty of speech
Poverty of content of speech
Catatonia
Stuperous state
Blunted affect
Anhedonia
Inappropriate affect
Avolition
Dementia praecox
Schizophrenia
Fundamental symptoms
First-rank symptoms
Thought broadcasting
Voices commenting
Somatic passivity
Schizophreniform disorders
Disorganized type
Catatonic type
Paranoid type
Undifferentiated type
Residual type
Type I syndrome
Type II syndrome
Schizoaffective disorder
Delusional disorder
Brief psychotic disorder
Prodromal phase
Residual phase
Lifetime morbid risk
Polygenic
Schizotaxia
High risk
Positron emission tomography (PET)

Neuroleptics
Dopamine hypothesis
Social causation hypothesis
Social selection hypothesis
Communication deviance
Index cases
Expressed emotion
Transactional
Vulnerability marker
Phenothiazines
Extrapyramidal symptoms
Tardive dyskinesia
Treatment resistance

KEY NAMES

The following individuals have made important contributions to the material presented in the chapter. Write out the names of these individuals and the theories, research, or treatment with which they are associated. Then check your answers with the information in your text.

Emil Kraeplin
Eugen Bleuler
Kurt Schneider
Robert Spitzer
Manfred Bleuler
Gregor Mendel
Irving Gottesman
Leonard Heston
Seymour Kety
Paul Meehl
Sarnoff Mednick
Daniel Weinberger
Lymann Wynne
Margaret Singer
Pekka Tienari
George Brown
John Wing
William Iacono
William Grove
Brett Clementz

MATCHING QUESTIONS

Match the following terms and names with the definitions presented below. The answers can be found at the end of the chapter.

a. prodromal phase
b. expressed emotion
c. Paul Meehl
d. perseveration
e. catatonia
f. vulnerability marker
g. dementia praecox
h. poverty of content of speech
i. residual phase
j. anhedonia

k. schizoaffective disorder
l. Kurt Schneider
m. neuroleptics
n. schizophreniform disorder
o. negative symptoms
p. tardive dyskinesia
q. lifetime morbid risk
r. schizophrenia
s. Irving Gottesman
t. derailment

1) _____ a term that refers to the inability to experience pleasure

2) _____ a type of communication deviance in which an individual speaks at length without conveying any meaningful information

3) _____ a psychologist who has made important contributions to our understanding of genetic factors in schizophrenia

4) _____ proposed that all indiviudals who are predisposed to schizophrenia inherit a type of subtle neurological defect, referred to as schizotaxia

5) _____ a term meaning the splitting of mental assocations

6) _____ an observable sign that indicates that a person is at risk for developing a particular disorder

7) _____ the proportion of a specific population that will be affected by a particular disorder at some point during their lives

8) _____ a type of disorder that is characterized by the combination of both schizophrenic and mood disorder symptoms

9) _____ another name for antipsychotic drugs

10) _____ a term coined by some individuals researching family interaction patterns in schizophrenia and referring to different types of negative or intrusive attitudes

11) _____ a German psychiatrist who developed a diagnostic system for schizophrenia based on his theory of "first-rank symptoms"

12) _____ following the active phase of schizophrenia, the individual may no longer be actively psychotic but continues to be impaired in various ways

13) _____ a term that means early and severe intellectual deterioration

14) _____ features of schizophrenia that presumably reflect the absence of normal functioning

15) _____ a type of motor disturbance characterized by immobility and marked muscular rigidity

16) _____ a type of verbal discommunication that involves persistently repeating the same word or phrase over and over again

17) _____ a syndrome caused by prolonged use of antipsychotic drugs and characterized by numerous abnormal involuntary movements

18) _____ a stage of schizophrenic disorder preceding the active phase and characterized by deterioration in role functioning

19) _____ a type of disorganized speech pattern in which the individual consistently shifts topics too abruptly

20) _____ a type of disorder in which schizophrenic-like symptoms are prominent for a period less than six months

MULTIPLE CHOICE QUESTIONS

The following multiple choice questions will test your comprehension of the material presented in the chapter. Circle the correct choice for each question in the section. Then compare your answers with those at the end of the chapter.

1) Which of the following would NOT be considered a positive symptom of schizophrenia?

    a. hallucinations
    b. blunted affect
    c. delusions
    d. disorganized speech

2) The distribution of schizophrenia within families is probably best explained by which of the following genetic models?

    a. polygenic
    b. single dominant gene
    c. single recessive gene
    d. linked genes

3) The trend in the DSM diagnosis of schizophrenia over time has been which of the following?

    a. include more affective symptoms
    b. omit subtyping of the disorder
    c. move from a broader to narrower definition of schizophrenia
    d. move from a more restrictive to less restrictive duration criterion

4) Research on the relationship between expressed emotion (EE) and schizophrenia supports which of the following?

    a. the presence of expressed emotion is only associated with the onset of an individual's initial episode of schizophrenia
    b. among the various types of comments that contribute to a high EE rating, criticism is typically most associated with the likelihood of relapse
    c. the influence of expressed emotions is unique to schizophrenia
    d. all of the above

5) A difference between schizophrenia and delusional disorder is that:

    a. patients with schizophrenia display less impairment in their daily functioning than patients with delusional disorder
    b. patients with delusional disorder display more negative symptoms during the active phase of their illness
    c. the behavior of patients with schizophrenia is considerably less bizarre
    d. patients with delusional disorder are preoccupied with delusions that are not necessarily considered bizarre

6) In the search to identify people who are vulnerable to schizophrenia, several potential vulnerability markers have been considered. Which of the following would NOT be considered a good criterion for a vulnerability marker?

    a. the marker should be able to distinguish between people who are already schizophrenic and people who are not
    b. the marker should be a characteristic which is stable over time
    c. the marker should be able to identify more people who are relatives of

schizophrenics than people in the general population
d. the marker should be able to predict the likelihood of relapse for
people who have already experienced their first episode of schizophrenia

7)   Research on schizophrenic twins and adopted-away offspring of schizophrenics suggests which of the following?

a. vulnerability to schizophrenia is consistently manifested by the same
symptoms of this disorder across relatives
b. vulnerability to schizophrenia is expressed through a variety of
different symptom patterns, including depressive and anxiety syndromes
c. vulnerability to schizophrenia is consistently manifested by the same
symptoms of this disorder only when male relatives are affected
d. vulnerability to schizophrenia is sometimes manifested by schizophrenialike
personality traits and non-schizophrenic psychotic disorders

8) Tangentiality is an example of which type of disturbance?

a. motor disturbance
b. affective disturbance
c. disorganized speech
d. delusional belief

9)   Which of the following statements is TRUE regarding the use of neuroleptic medication?

a. beneficial effects are noticed within 24 hours after beginning
neuroleptic medication
b. neurolopetic drugs appear to be particularly effective for relief of the
positive symptoms associated with schizophrenia
c. almost all schizophrenic patients are considered to be complete
responders to this type of medication
d. schizophrenic patients with the most severe symptoms appear to respond
best to neuroleptic drugs

10) Individuals who exhibit psychotic symptoms for no more than a month and that cannot be attributed to other disorders such as substance abuse or mood disorder usually receive the diagnosis of:

a. delusional disorder
b. schizophreniform disorder
c. brief psychotic disorder
d. schizoaffective disorder

11) Which of the following is NOT a possible explanation for the relationship between the presence of familial communication problems and schizophrenia?

    a. parental communication problems may cause the child's disorder
    b. the child's adjustment problems may cause the parents' problems
    c. both the child's disorder and the parent communication problems reflect
       a common genetic influence
    d. all of the above are possible explanations for the presence of this relationship

12) Which of the following reflects a change in the DSM-IV definition of schizophrenia:

    a. negative symptoms assume a more prominent role
    b. positive symptoms assume a more prominent role
    c. the person must display active symptoms of the illness for at least one year
    d. a decline in the person's functioning is no longer required

13) An interesting and consistent result across numerous CT scan studies has been that:

    a. some people with schizophrenia have an enlarged hypothalamus
    b. some people with schizophrenia have enlarged lateral ventricles
    c. some people with schizophrenia have enlarged temporal lobes
    d. some people with schizophrenia have a reduced amount of cerebrospinal fluid

14) A restriction of an individual's nonverbal display of his or her emotional responses is referred to as:

    a. blunted affect
    b. affective loosening
    c. anhedonia
    d. inappropriate affect

15) Studies investigating the relationship between social class and schizophrenia support that risk for the disorder:

    a. is associated with adverse social and economic circumstances
    b. is not associated by circumstances most likely to be present in the
       lives of people who are economically disadvantaged
    c. is associated with the unique types of circumstances most frequently
       affiliated with high social class
    d. is most associated with recent immigration to a country

16) Which statement about the course of schizophrenia is TRUE?

    a. a significant amount of individuals experience their first episode between 35-50 years of age

b. the onset of the disorder typically occurs during adolescence or early adulthood

c. the active phase of illness is always the longest of the three phases

d. the premorbid phase of illness usually lasts no longer than six months

17) Inconsistencies associated with the dopamine model of schizophrenia include which of the following?

a. dopamine blockage begins immediately when medication is administered but the drugs often take several days to become effective

b. some patients do not respond positively to drugs that block dopamine receptors

c. studies investigating the byproducts of dopamin in cerebrospinal fluid are inconsisent and inconclusive

d. all of the above

18) Which of the following is NOT included in the DSM-IV as a subtype of schizophrenia?

a. paranoid

b. residual

c. undifferentiated

d. negative

19) The Danish high-risk for schizophrenia project has supported which of the following hypotheses?

a. families with individuals who develop the positive symptoms of the disorder appear to be at higher genetic risk

b. children who experience head injuries before age five appear to be at greater risk for schizophrenia

c. neurodevelopmental problems in schizophrenia are antecedents rather than consequences of the disorder

d. problems in delivery at birth do not appear to be associated with vulnerability to schizophrenia

20) A criticism of twin studies and their persuasive evidence for the role of genetic factors in schizophrenia is that:

a. DZ and MZ twin concordance rates are approximately equal, suggesting that genetic factors are actually less important than environmental factors

b. MZ twins, because of their physical similarity, are probably treated more similarly by their parents than even DZ twins, which confounds environmental with genetic factors

c. the studies determining concordance rates are flawed because they do not take into account the birth order of the MZ twins

d. the concordance rates for MZ twins for schizophrenia has fluctuated dramatically across studies

21) The potentially exciting part of eye-tracking dysfunction and the possibility of this characteristic being a vulnerability marker for schizophrenia is that:

a. eye-tracking dysfunction appears to be influenced by genetic factors and is apparently a stable trait

b. eye-tracking dysfunction appears to be present only in patients with schizophrenia

c. approximately 90% of the first-degree relatives of schizophrenic individuals show this characteristic

d. the eye-tracking dysfunction only manifests itself during episodes of schizophrenia

22) Joe's behavior has been observed on the hospital ward for several hours. He has been sitting perfectly still in one position. Furthermore, he has been completely mute (has not spoken a single word) since admission. Which subtype of schizophrenia best represents Joe's behavior?

a. disorganized
b. paranoid
c. catatonic
d. undifferentiated

23) Research suggests that the outcome of schizophrenia may be best described by which of the following statements?

a. 50% of the individuals continue to deteriorate after their first episode, 10% completely recover, and 40% experience intermittent episodes

b. 30% of the individuals recover fairly well after their initial episode, 30% continue to deteriorate, and 40% continue to experience intermittent episodes

c. approximately 60% of the individuals recover fairly well after their initial episode, while 40% continue to deteriorate

d. approximately 60% of the individuals continue to deteriorate after their initial episode, while 40% continue to experience intermittent episodes

24) When Samuel grins as he talks about the loss of his father in a traumatic accident, he is displaying:

a. disorganized affect
b. avolition

c. catatonia

d. inappropriate affect

25) The theory that harmful events associated with being a member of the lowest social class (e.g., poor nutrition, social isolation) is called:

    a. the social class hypothesis

    b. the social causation hypothesis

    c. the social impairment hypothesis

    d. the social selection hypothesis

26) The usefulness of subtyping schizophrenia has been criticized because:

    a. some individuals do not fit the traditional subtype descriptions

    b. some individuals display the symptoms of more than one subtype simultaneously

    c. the symptoms of some individuals change from one episode to the next, reflecting subtype instability

    d. all of the above

27) The average concordance rate for monozygotic twins for schizophrenia is:

    a. 22%

    b. 36%

    c. 48%

    d. 72%

28) Perhaps the most unpleasant side effect associated with the use of neuroleptics is:

    a. the fact that the drugs must be taken for two to four months before the patient experiences relief from symptoms

    b. potentially toxic reactions to the drugs if the patient's diet is not carefully monitored

    c. the presence of extrapyramidal symptoms

    d. acute gastrointestinal symptoms (e.g., nausea, vomiting) during the first few weeks of use

29) Research on gender differences in schizophrenia supports that:

    a. men experience their first episode of schizophrenia about five years later than women

    b. women typically display better premorbid social competence prior to their first episode of schizophrenia

    c. men typically display a less chronic course compared to women

    d. women display more negative symptoms

30) Bleuler's definition of schizophrenia emphasized which of the following?

    a. signs and symptoms of the disorder
    b. course and outcome
    c. genetic vulnerability markers
    d. impairment in social roles

BRIEF ESSAY

As a final exercise, write out answers to the following brief essay questions. Then compare your answers with the material presented in the text.

After you have answered these questions, review the "Critical Thinking" questions that are presented at the end of the text chapter. Answering these questions will help you integrate important issues and themes that have been featured throughout the chapter.

1. Pretend that you are on the committee that will be responsible for developing the definition for schizophrenia (i.e., the diagnostic criteria) for DSM-V. Signs and symptoms, duration of episodes, degree of impairment, familial, biological, genetic data, etc.- what would you consider to be the most appropriate criteria to be included in your definition and why?

2. Explain what is meant by the diathesis-stress model of schizophrenia. Which factors reviewed in your text would represent the diathesis? Which factors would represent stress?

3. Review the questions and considerations that an investigator must address as s/he designs a research project in psychopathology, comparing patients with a certain diagnosis with a comparison group. What are the issues involved in the selection of a meaningful comparison group?

4. Briefly describe and compare the three forms of psychosocial treatment reviewed in your textbook that have been shown to be effective for schizophrenia. What are their advantages and disadvantages as treatment programs?

ANSWER KEY

MATCHING EXERCISES

1. j	11. l
2. h	12. i
3. s	13. g
4. c	14. o
5. r	15. e
6. f	16. d
7. q	17. p
8. k	18. a
9. m	19. t
10. b	20. n

MULTIPLE CHOICE EXERCISES

1. b	6. d	11. d
2. a	7. d	12. a
3. c	8. c	13. b
4. b	9. b	14. a
5. d	10. c	15. a

16. b	21. a	26. d
17. d	22. c	27. c
18. d	23. b	28. c
19. c	24. d	29. b
20. b	25. b	30. a

CHAPTER THIRTEEN
DEMENTIA, DELIRIUM, AND AMNESTIC DISORDERS

CHAPTER OUTLINE

Overview

Dementia: Typical Symptoms and Associated Features
    Cognitive Symptoms
        Memory and Learning
        Verbal Communication
        Perception
        Abstract Thinking
    Assessment of Cognitive Impairment
    Associated Features
        Emotion
        Motor Behavior
        Psychotic Symptoms

Amnestic Disorder: Typical Symptoms and Associated Features
    Brief Historical Perspective
    Diagnostic and Statistical Manual of Mental Disorders (DSM-IV)
    Specific Disorders
        Dementia of the Alzheimer's Type
        Pick's Disease
        Huntington's Disease
        Parkinson's Disease
        Vascular Dementia
        Dementia versus Depression

Epidemiology
    Incidence and Prevalence by Age Groups

Etiological Considerations and Research
    Genetic Factors
    Neurotransmitters
    Viral Infections
    Immune System Dysfunction
    Environmental Factors

Treatment and Management
    Medication
    Environmental and Behavioral Management
    Support for Caregivers

Summary

LEARNING OBJECTIVES

After reviewing the material presented in this chapter, you should be able to:

*   define and distinguish dementia, delirium, and amnestic disorders

*   distinguish retrograde from anterograde amnesia

*   describe the primary symptoms of aphasia, apraxia, and agnosia

*   identify the functions of neuropsychological assessment in the diagnosis
        of dementia

*   describe some of the primary features of amnestic disorder and distinguish them
        from dementia

*   identify the key contributions of Pinel, Broca, Wernicke, Korsakoff,
        Alzheimer, and Kraepelin in the diagnosis of cognitive disorders

*   distinguish primary from secondary dementia--and differentiated from
        undifferentiated primary dementia

*   describe some of the features of Alzheimer's, Pick's, Huntington's, Parkinson's, and
        vascular diseases

*   describe the role of genetics, neurotransmitters, viral infections, and
        environmental factors in the development of cognitive disorders

*   know the importance of accurate diagnosis in the treatment of dementia

*   discuss the importance of environmental and behavioral management as well
        as caregiver support and respite programs in treatment of the patient suffering from
        a cognitive disorder

KEY TERMS AND CONCEPTS

Following is a list of key terms and concepts that are featured in the chapter and are important for you to know. Write out the definitions of each of these terms and check your answers with the definitions in the text.

Dementia
Delirium

Amnestic disorders
Cognitive disorders
Neurologists
Acquired disorder
Retrograde amnesia
Anterograde amnesia
Cognitive mechanics
Cognitive pragmatics
Selective optimization with compensation
Aphasia
Apraxia
Agnosia
Neuropsychological assessment
Primary dementia
Secondary dementia
Undifferentiated primary dementia
Differentiated primary dementia
Alzheimer's disease
Explicit memory
Implicit memory
Neurofibrillary tangles
Senile plaques
Pick's disease
Huntington's disease
Parkinson's disease
Substantia nigra
Vascular dementia
Multi-infarct dementia
Pseudodementia
Autosomal dominant trait
Genetic linkage
Chromosome marker
Restriction fragment length polymorphisms (RFLPs)
Creutzfeldt-Jakob disease
Acetylcholine (ACH)
Choline acetyl transferase
Respite programs

KEY NAMES

The following individuals have made important contributions to the material presented in the chapter. Write out the names of these individuals and the theories, research, or treatment with which they are associated. Then check your answers with the information in your text.

Paul Baltes
Phillip Pinel
Paul Broca
Carl Wernicke
Syergey Korsakoff
Alois Alzheimer
Emil Kraepelin
Thomas Hunt Morgan

MATCHING QUESTIONS

Match the following terms and names with the definitions presented below. The answers can be found at the end of the chapter.

a. agnosia
b. Korsakoff's syndrome
c. Paul Broca
d. implicit memory
e. senile plaques
f. Pick's bodies
g. primary dementia
h. multi-infarct dementia
i. apraxia
j. retrograde amnesia

k. anterograde amnesia
l. a stroke
m. pseudodementia
n. secondary dementia
o. Creutzfeldt-Jakob disease
p. neurofibrils
q. Phillip Pinel
r. explicit memory
s. infarct
t. aphasia

1) _____ refers to the loss of memory for events prior to the onset of an illness or the experience of a traumatic event

2) _____ refers to the area of dead tissue produced by a stroke

3) _____ also referred to as declarative memory

4) _____ dementia in which the cognitive impairment is produced by the direct effect of a disease on brain tissue

5) _____ French surgeon who demonstrated that a specific type of aphasia is associated with lesions in the left frontal lobe

165

6) _____   consists of a central core of homogeneous protein material surrounded by clumps of debris left over from destroyed neurons

7) _____   also known as vascular dementia

8) _____   an example of an infection that develops over a much more extended period of time than do most viral infections

9) _____   describes various types of loss or impairment in language that are a result of brain damage

10) _____   condition of patients with symptoms of dementia whose cognitive impairment is actually produced by a major depressive disorder

11) _____   technically means "perception without meaning", and refers to difficulties in identifying stimuli in the environment

12) _____   a distinctive ballooning of nerve cells

13) _____   refers to the severe interruption of blood flow to the brain

14) _____   provides structural support for the cell and help transport chemicals that are used in the production of neurotransmitters

15) _____   subject's performance on this type of memory task may be enhanced by prior experience with the target information

16) _____   dementia in which cognitive impairment is a byproduct or side effect of some other type of biological or psychological dysfunction

17) _____   an alcohol-induced persisting amnestic disorder

18) _____   a psychiatrist who provided the first modern descriptions of dementia

19) _____   refers to the inability to learn or to remember new material after a particular point in time

20) _____   difficulty performing purposeful movements in response to verbal commands

MULTIPLE CHOICE QUESTIONS

The following multiple choice questions will test your comprehension of the material presented in the chapter. Circle the correct choice for each question in the section. Then compare your answers with those at the end of the chapter.

1) All of the following are goals in designing an environment conducive to demented patients EXCEPT:

    a. keep the patients relatively inactive in order to prevent them from hurting themselves
    b. facilitate the patients knowledge of the environment through labeled rooms, hallways, etc.
    c. keep the environment negotiable (i.e., keep areas that a person will use often visible from their room if they cannot be remembered)
    d. stay abreast of safety and health issues

2) _____ is a type of motor dysfunction that involves jerky, semi-purposeful movements of the person's face and limbs.

    a. Anoxia
    b. Myotonia
    c. Chorea
    d. Lipofuscin

3) A German neurologist who identified a form of aphasia seen in patients with damage to the posterior cortex.

    a. Syergey Korsakoff
    b. Carl Wernicke
    c. Alois Alzheimer
    d. Emil Kraepelin

4) All of the following are typical symptoms of Parkinson's disease EXCEPT:

    a. tremors
    b. postural abnormalities
    c. gradual dementia
    d. reduction in voluntary movements

5) A _____ deals primarily with diseases of the brain and the nervous system.

    a. neurologist

b. psychiatrist

c. psychologist

d. cardiologist

6) Which of the following diagnoses depends on the presence of a positive family history for the disorder?

a. Parkinson's disease

b. Alzheimer's disease

c. Pick's disease

d. Huntington's disease

7) According to Paul Baltes, _____ is to fluid intelligence as _____ is to crystallized intelligence.

a. wisdom; knowledge

b. knowledge; wisdom

c. cognitive mechanics; cognitive pragmatics

d. cognitive pragmatics; cognitive mechanics

8) The _____ is probably the best known neuropsychological assessment procedure that involves the examination of performance on psychological tests to indicate whether a person has a brain disorder.

a. Halstead-Reitan

b. Weschler

c. Symptoms Checklist-90 (SCL-90)

d. Minnesota Multiphasic Personality Inventory-2 (MMPI-2)

9) The DSM-IV currently classifies dementia and related clinical phenomena as:

a. organic mental disorders

b. biological mental disorders

c. psychological disorders with organic etiology

d. cognitive disorders

10) Hallucinations and delusions are seen in about _____ of dementia cases.

a. 10%

b. 20%

c. 30%

d. 40%

11) The most effective form of treatment for improving cognitive functioning in dementia of the Alzheimer's type is:

    a. cognitive therapy
    b. cognitive-behavioral therapy
    c. rational-emotive therapy (RET)
    d. no form of treatment is presently capable of improving cognitive
       functioning in dementia of the Alzheimer's type

12) One theory regarding the condition of Korsakoff's syndrome suggests that lack of _____ leads to atrophy of the medial thalamus.

    a. zinc
    b. vitamin C
    c. vitamin B1 (thiamin)
    d. potassium

13) Which of the following is a confusional state that develops over a short period of time and is often associated with agitation and hyperactivity:

    a. delirium
    b. amnesia
    c. dementia
    d. Alzheimer's disease

14) Betty's physician presented her with a hairbrush and said "show me what you do with this object." Betty took the brush and brushed her hair with it, but was unable to name the object. Betty is most likely suffering from which of the following?

    a. agnosia
    b. aphasia
    c. apraxia
    d. ataxia

15) All of the following are frequently associated with dementia EXCEPT:

    a. personality changes
    b. emotional difficulties
    c. high frequency of drug abuse
    d. motivational problems

16) A definite diagnosis of Alzheimer's disease requires the observation of:

    a. neurofibrillary tangles and senile plaques

b. degeneration of the substantia nigra

c. enlargement of the hypothalamus

d. all of the above

17) Which of the following transmitters has been shown to have reduced levels in Alzheimer's patients?

a. acetylcholine (Ach)

b. serotonin

c. norepinephrine

d. dopamine

18) In order to qualify for a diagnosis of dementia, the person must exhibit memory impairment and which of the following?

a. aggressive behavior

b. problems in abstract thinking

c. at least one previous episode of delirium

d. age of at least 65 years

19) All of the following are true of delirium EXCEPT:

a. it usually has a rapid onset

b. speech is typically confused

c. the person usually remains alert and responsive to the environment

d. it can be resolved

20) Parkinson's disease is primarily a disorder of the motor system that is caused by a loss of the neurotransmitter dopamine and a degeneration of this specific area of the brain stem:

a. substantia nigra

b. thalamus

c. fornix

d. superior colliculi

21) Although controversial, epidemiologic investigations have discovered that some types of dementia, especially Alzheimer's disease, may be related to all of the following EXCEPT:

a. aluminum

b. cigarette smoking

c. level of educational experience

d. lead

22) The incidence of dementia will be much greater in the near future because:

a. diagnostic criteria are more loosely defined

b. the average age of the population is increasing steadily

c. more people are being exposed to the environmental factors that have
   been shown to cause dementia

d. dementia is now striking people at a much earlier age

23) Which of the following can be distinguished from other types of dementia listed in the DSM-IV on the basis of speed of onset (i.e., cognitive impairment appears gradually, and the person's cognitive deterioration is progressive)?

a. vascular dementia

b. Huntington's disease

c. Alzheimer's disease

d. substance-induced persisting dementia

24) Which of the following is an example of a differentiated dementia?

a. Huntington's disease

b. Alzheimer's disease

c. vascular dementia

d. HIV disease

25) _____ is a disorder that is frequently associated with dementia.

a. Bipolar disorder

b. Depression

c. Schizophrenia

d. Multiple personality disorder

26) Some studies have confirmed an association between Alzheimer's disease and which of the following:

a. dependent personality disorder

b. vascular dementia

c. Korsakoff's syndrome

d. Down syndrome

27) Which of the following is/are treatment options for demented patients?

a. behavioral strategies

b. cognitive strategies

c. insight-oriented strategies

d. all of the above

171

28) Almost _____ of people over 90 years of age exhibit symptoms of moderate or severe dementia.

     a. 25%
     b. 40%
     c. 65%
     d. 80%

29) All of the following are true of delirium EXCEPT:

     a. it typically fluctuates throughout the day and is usually worse at night
     b. the delirious person loses the ability to learn new information or becomes unable to recall previously learned information
     c. the delirious person is likely to be disoriented with relation to time or place
     d. the primary symptom is clouding of consciousness, which might also be described as a person's reduced awareness of his or her surroundings

30) Which of the following appears to be the most common type of dementia?

     a. Pick's disease
     b. Huntington's disease
     c. Alzheimer's disease
     d. vascular dementia

BRIEF ESSAY

As a final exercise, write out answers to the following brief essay questions. Then compare your answers with the material presented in the text.

After you have answered these questions, review the "Critical Thinking" questions that are presented at the end of the text chapter. Answering these questions will help you integrate important issues and themes that have been featured throughout the chapter.

1. Briefly discuss how the behavioral effects of a stroke are different from those of dementia.

2. Discuss the environmental factors that have been shown to be possibly linked to some types of dementia. What do you see as being problematic with these findings? What must we be cautious of when interpreting this data?

3. Briefly discuss the similarities and differences between dementia and depression. Discuss a case where it might be difficult to distinguish them apart. How could this be done?

4. Briefly review the defining characteristics of delirium, Korsakoff's syndrome, Alzheimer's disease, and Huntington's disease.

ANSWER KEY

MATCHING EXERCISES

1. j	11. a
2. s	12. f
3. r	13. l
4. g	14. p
5. c	15. d
6. e	16. n
7. h	17. b
8. o	18. q
9. t	19. k
10. m	20. i

MULTIPLE CHOICE EXERCISES

1. a	6. d	11. d
2. c	7. c	12. c
3. b	8. a	13. a
4. c	9. d	14. b
5. a	10. b	15. c

16. d	21. d	26. d
17. a	22. b	27. d
18. b	23. c	28. b
19. c	24. a	29. b
20. a	25. b	30. c

CHAPTER FOURTEEN
MENTAL RETARDATION and PERVASIVE DEVELOPMENT DISORDERS

CHAPTER OUTLINE

Overview

Mental Retardation
> Typical Symptoms and Associated Features
>> Limitations in Adaptive Skills
>> Onset in Developmental Period
> Classification
>> Brief Historical Perspective
>> Contemporary Classification
> Epidemiology
> Etiological Considerations and Research
>> Biological Factors
>>> Chromosomal Disorders
>>> Genetic Disorders
>>> Infectious Diseases
>>> Toxins
>>> Other Biological Abnormalities
>>> Normal Genetic Variation
>> Psychological Factors
>> Social Factors
> Treatment: Primary, Secondary, and Tertiary Prevention and Normalization
>> Primary Prevention
>> Secondary Prevention
>> Tertiary Prevention
>> Normalization

Autism and Pervasive Developmental Disorders
> Typical Symptoms and Associated Features
>> Impaired Social Interaction
>> Impaired Communication
>> Stereotyped Behavior, Interests, and Activities
>> Apparent Sensory Deficits
>> Self-injury
>> Savant Performance
> Classification
>> Brief Historical Perspective
>> Contemporary Classification
> Epidemiology

LEARNING OBJECTIVES

After reviewing the material presented in this chapter, you should be able to:

* identify the basic defining characteristics of mental retardation and autism

* distinguish between practical intelligence and social intelligence

* identify the four levels of mental retardation that DSM-IV delineates: mild, moderate, severe, and profound

* appreciate that mental retardation can be caused by a variety of biological factors: chromosomal disorders, genetic disorders, infectious diseases, and environmental or chemical toxins

* distinguish between primary, secondary, and tertiary prevention in the treatment of mental retardation

* describe the types of difficulties autistic children have with social interactions

* define dysprosody, echolalia, and pronoun reversal as they apply to impaired communication in autism

* know the basic epidemiological statistics for autism

* provide five reasons supporting the current belief that autism is a biologically-based disorder

* understand the advantages and disadvantages of intensive behavior modification treatment for autism

KEY TERMS AND CONCEPTS

Following is a list of key terms and concepts that are featured in the chapter and are important for you to know. Write out the definitions of each of these terms and check your answers with the definitions in the text.

Mental retardation
Intelligence quotient (IQ)
Practical intelligence
Social intelligence
Intensity of needed support
Mild mental retardation
Moderate mental retardation
Severe mental retardation
Profound mental retardation
Down syndrome
Trisomy 21
Fragile-X-syndrome
Klinefelter syndrome
XYY syndrome
Turner syndrome
Phenylketonuria (PKU)
Phenylalanine
Phenylalanine hydroxylase
Tuberous sclerosis
Tay-sachs disease
Hurler syndrome (Gargoylism)
Lesch-Nyhan syndrome
Cytomegalovirus
Toxoplasmosis
Rubella
Syphilis
Genital herpes
Encephalitis
Meningitis
Fetal alcohol syndrome
Crack babies
Mercury poisoning
Lead poisoning
Rh incompatibility
Premature birth
Asphyxia

Malnutrition
Epilepsy
Cultural-familial retardation
Heritability ratios
Amniocentesis
Respite care
Normalization
Mainstreaming
Deinstitutionalization movement
Pervasive developmental disorders
Autism
Gaze aversion
Dysprosody
Echolalia
Pronoun reversal
Self-stimulation
Apparent sensory deficit
Self-injurious behavior
Savant performance
Asperger's disorder
Eidectic imagery
Childhood disintegrative disorder
Developmental aphasia
"Refrigerator parents"
Experimental hypothesis
Null hypothesis
Epistemology
Fenfluramine
Plasticity
Facilitated communication

KEY NAMES

The following individuals have made important contributions to the material presented in the chapter. Write out the names of these individuals and the theories, research, or treatment with which they are associated. Then check your answers with the information in your text.

Alfred Binet
Jean Marc Itard
Langdon Down
Leo Kanner
Hans Asperger

Rosemary Crossley
Douglas Biklen
O. Ivar Lovaas

MATCHING QUESTIONS

Match the following terms and names with the definitions presented below. The answers can be found at the end of the chapter.

a. practical intelligence
b. dysprosody
c. Turner syndrome
d. autism
e. amniocentesis
f. intelligence quotient
g. Klinefelter syndrome
h. toxoplasmosis
i. cultural-familial retardation
j. social intelligence

k. Asperger's disorder
l. null hypothesis
m. childhood disintegrative disorder
n. O. Ivar Lovaas
o. Hurler syndrome
p. pervasive developmental disorder
q. Jean Marc Itard
r. developmental aphasia
s. facilitated communication
t. experimental hypothesis

1) _____ characterized by the presence of one or more extra X chromosomes in males

2) _____ a disorder characterized by delayed or absent speech

3) _____ in experimental procedures, the hypothesis of "no difference"

4) _____ describes unusual subtleties of speaking style (i.e., speech production is disturbed in its rate, rhythm, and intonation)

5) _____ a protozoan infection during pregnancy, which is contracted from ingestion of infected raw meats or from contact with infected cat feces

6) _____ a measure of an individual's intellectual ability

7) _____ a technique in which the hand and arm of a disabled individual is supported, thus allowing the individual to communicate through a keyboard

8) _____ also referred to as gargoylism, this results in gross physical abnormalities including dwarfism, humpback, a bulging head, and clawlike hands

9) _____ a psychologist who is an acknowledged leader in applying behavior modification techniques for autistic children

10) _____ dictionaries often define this as "absorption in one's own mental activity"

11) _____ refers to the ability to manage the ordinary activities of daily living

12) _____ this individual was instrumental in spurring efforts to develop special education programs for the mentally retarded

13) _____ an umbrella classification that includes autism and autistic-like disorders that fail to meet the criteria for autism

14) _____ the hypothesis predicted by the investigator given that certain conditions are met or certain variables manipulated

15) _____ cases of mental retardation of unknown etiology

16) _____ onset of this disorder occurs after at least 2 years of normal development and is characterized by problems in social interaction and communication, in addition to stereotyped behavior

17) _____ a disorder that is identical to autism, with the exception that the disorder involves no clinically significant delay in language

18) _____ a diagnostic procedure in which fluid is extracted from the sac that protects the fetus during pregnancy

19) _____ referred to as the XO configuration in females, girls with this are typically small, fail to develop sexually, and generally have intelligence near or within the normal range

20) _____ refers to the ability to understand how to conduct yourself in social situations

MULTIPLE CHOICE QUESTIONS

The following multiple choice questions will test your comprehension of the material presented in the chapter. Circle the correct choice for each question in the section. Then compare your answers with those at the end of the chapter.

1) Which of the following toxins presents the greatest threat to a fetus?

    a. cigarettes
    b. alcohol
    c. lead
    d. mercury

2) All of the following are central symptoms of autism EXCEPT:

    a. impaired communication abilities
    b. impairments in social interaction
    c. abnormalities of the eyes, nose, and ears
    d. stereotyped patterns of behavior, interests, and activities

3) Mild mental retardation is designated for individuals with IQ scores between which of the following?

    a. 20-25 and 40
    b. 35-40 and 50
    c. 50-55 and 70
    d. 65-70 and 90

4) As outlined in your text, which of the following has been suggested as an interpretation for pronoun reversal as documented in some cases of autism?

    a. pronoun reversal demonstrates a lack of understanding of speech
    b. pronoun reversal is a result of faulty neurotransmitters
    c. pronoun reversal results from damage to specific areas in the frontal lobe
    d. pronoun reversal is due to the autistic child's disinterest in other people

5) Autism is considered to be a _____ disorder, with approximately _____ out of every 10,000 children qualifying for the diagnosis.

    a. rare; 4-5
    b. rare; 20-25
    c. common; 1,000-1,500
    d. common; 3,000-3,500

6) Which of the following is one of the most important current secondary prevention efforts in preventing cultural-familial retardation?

    a. amniocentesis
    b. prenatal care
    c. Head Start

d. respite care

7) Treatment for self-injurious behavior that is sometimes seen in autistic children is controversial because:

    a. there is no empirical support to back up the treatment
    b. the treatment typically involves punishment (e.g., slap or mild electric shock)
    c. the treatment has been relatively ineffective
    d. the treatment has been used without guardian consent

8) The reaction range concept of IQ proposed that (the) _____ determines the upper and lower limits of IQ, and (the) _____ determines the extent to which people fulfill their genetic potential.

    a. heredity; experience
    b. experience; heredity
    c. parents' IQ; age
    d. age; parents' IQ

9) Mental retardation with a specific, known organic cause:

    a. is typically more common among families living in poverty
    b. generally is more common among Hispanics and African-Americans
    c. is most prevalent among the upper class
    d. generally has an equal prevalence among all social classes

10) Which of the following was the original developer of IQ tests?

    a. Douglas Biklen
    b. Alfred Binet
    c. Leo Kanner
    d. Rosemary Crossley

11) All of the following are true of autistic children EXCEPT:

    a. most are normal in physical appearance
    b. physical growth and development is generally normal
    c. their body movements are typically grossly uncoordinated
    d. they sometimes have unusual actions and postures

12) Premature birth is defined either as a birth weight of less than 5 1/2 pounds or as birth before _____ weeks of gestation.

    a. 35

b. 36
c. 37
d. 38

13) The most common form of self-injury that can accompany autism and other pervasive developmental disorders is:

a. head-banging
b. repetitive hitting of objects with one's fists
c. dare-devil behaviors (i.e., skydiving, bungee jumping, etc.)
d. cutting of oneself with sharp objects

14) Which of the following "intensity of needed support" levels is characterized by regular involvement (e.g., daily) in at least some environments (such as work or home) and not time-limited (e.g., long-term support and long-term home living support)?

a. intermittent
b. limited
c. extensive
d. pervasive

15) Autism is believed to be caused by:

a. poor parenting
b. an abusive environment
c. neurological abnormalities
d. there is no known etiology for autism

16) Almost _____ of all children in the United States are born to adolescent mothers.

a. 8%
b. 12%
c. 16%
d. 20%

17) All of the following are diagnostic criteria for autism EXCEPT:

a. lack of social or emotional reciprocity
b. a prior diagnosis of Rett's disorder
c. apparently compulsive adherence to specific, nonfunctional routines or rituals
d. lack of varied spontaneous make-believe play or social imitative play
   appropriate to developmental level

18) Savant performance typically involves all of the following areas EXCEPT:

    a. artistic
    b. mathematical
    c. musical
    d. athletic

19) Which of the following interpretations of self-stimulation is most plausible according to your text?

    a. self-stimulation is a way for the autistic child to feel like he or she is similar to others
    b. self-stimulation serves the purpose of increasing stimulation to the autistic child who receives too little sensory input
    c. self-stimulation serves the function of making a terrifying world more constant and predictable and therefore less frightening
    d. self-stimulation is merely a repetitive behavior that serves no function

20) According to the American Association on Mental Retardation's (AAMR) definition, mental retardation manifests before age:

    a. 5
    b. 8
    c. 13
    d. 18

21) Which of the following is an infectious disease that is the result of infection of the brain and produces inflammation and permanent damage in approximately 20% of all cases?

    a. meningitis
    b. rubella
    c. encephalitis
    d. cytomegalovirus

22) Which of the following is caused by the presence of an extra chromosome and is characterized by a distinctively abnormal physical appearance, which includes slanting eyes, small head and stature, protruding tongue, and a variety of organ, muscle, and skeletal abnormalities?

    a. Down syndrome
    b. Fetal Alcohol syndrome
    c. Phenylketonuria (PKU)
    d. Tuberous sclerosis

23) Severe mental retardation accounts for approximately _____ of the mentally retarded.

    a. 1-2%
    b. 3-4%
    c. 8-10%
    d. 12-15%

24) Which of the following is the most promising approach to treating autism?

    a. intensive behavior modification using operant conditioning techniques
    b. antidepressant medication
    c. psychodynamic therapy that focuses on providing a nurturing, supportive environment
    d. none of the above have been effective in treating autism

25) Both mental retardation and pervasive developmental disorders include all of the following EXCEPT:

    a. either are present at birth or begin early in life
    b. serious disruptions in many areas of functioning, often including an inability to care for oneself independently
    c. gross physical abnormalities
    d. often, but not always, associated with a below-average IQ

26) Autism is usually first noticed:

    a. early in life
    b. during the teenage years
    c. in adulthood
    d. late in life

27) Which of the following terms was used for several years to classify autism together with other severe forms of childhood psychopathology?

    a. childhood dissociation
    b. disruptive childhood behaviors
    c. psychopathology first evident in childhood
    d. childhood schizophrenia

28) Which of the following developmental periods is particularly important to the course of autism?

    a. birth to 6 months

b. 6 - 36 months

c. early school years

d. early adulthood

29) Chase is a 6-year-old male who has been diagnosed with autism. Frequently, when asked "would you like a drink", Chase will repeat the question over and over again. This is an example of:

a. pronoun reversal

b. dysprosody

c. echolalia

d. self-stimulation

30) A(n) _____ environment is one that challenges children's developing intellectual skills and a(n) _____ environment offers encouragement for their pursuits.

a. responsive; stimulating

b. stimulating; responsive

c. adaptive; enriched

d. enriched; adaptive

BRIEF ESSAY

As a final exercise, write out answers to the following brief essay questions. Then compare your answers with the material presented in the text.

After you have answered these questions, review the "Critical Thinking" questions that are presented at the end of the text chapter. Answering these questions will help you integrate important issues and themes that have been featured throughout the chapter.

1. Despite the value of IQ tests in predicting academic performance, one controversial question is whether intelligence tests are "culture fair." Briefly discuss your views on this topic, including material from your chapter to support your ideas.

2. Currently, mental retardation can be classified according to the American Association on Mental Retardation (AAMR) and by the DSM-IV. Briefly discuss the similarities and differences in classification according to these two approaches.

3. Briefly discuss the various etiological considerations regarding autism. Which hypotheses seem most plausible to you and why? What research supports these hypotheses?

4. Briefly discuss the ethical debate regarding behavior modification treatments for decreasing potentially dangerous behaviors in autistic children. Do you believe these treatments to be unethical? If so, what do you believe are some viable options?

ANSWER KEY

MATCHING EXERCISES

1. g	11. a
2. r	12. q
3. l	13. p
4. b	14. t
5. h	15. i
6. f	16. m
7. s	17. k
8. o	18. e
9. n	19. c
10. d	20. j

MULTIPLE CHOICE EXERCISES

1. b	6. c	11. c
2. c	7. b	12. d
3. c	8. a	13. a
4. a	9. d	14. c
5. a	10. b	15. c

16. a	21. c	26. a
17. b	22. a	27. d
18. d	23. b	28. c
19. c	24. a	29. c
20. d	25. c	30. b

CHAPTER FIFTEEN
PSYCHOLOGICAL PROBLEMS OF CHILDHOOD AND EATING DISORDERS

CHAPTER OUTLINE

Overview

LEARNING OBJECTIVES

After reviewing the material presented in this chapter, you should be able to:

*   distinguish between externalizing and internalizing disorders of childhood

*   state some of the primary factors considered in the evaluation of externalizing symptoms

*   compare separation anxiety with separation anxiety disorder

*   understand that children's psychological problems are not simply miniature versions of adult disorders

*   describe some of the rare childhood disorders such as Pica, Rumination disorder, Tourette's disorder, Selective mutism, Reactive attachment disorder, Stereotypic movement disorder, Encopresis, and Enurisis

*   give the defining characteristics of conduct disorder, oppositional defiant disorder, and attention-deficit/hyperactivity disorder

*   understand how attachment theory attempts to explain disorders of childhood

*   state and describe the four parenting styles and explain how inconsistent parenting leads to externalizing symptoms in children

*   list and describe some of the genetic and biological evidence, both positive and negative, concerning etiology of disorders of childhood

*   describe the ways in which behavioral family therapy is utilized in the treatment of externalizing disorders

*   define binges and purges as they are used in the diagosis of eating disorders

*   identify the primary features of anorexia nervosa and bulimia nervosa

*   provide evidence of the effect of culture on the prevalence of eating disorders

*   describe the basic treatment approaches and the expected outcomes for anorexia nervosa and bulimia nervosa

KEY TERMS AND CONCEPTS

Following is a list of key terms and concepts that are featured in the chapter and are important for you to know. Write out the definitions of each of these terms and check your answers with the definitions in the text.

Externalizing disorders
Attention-deficit/hyperactivity disorder
Oppositional defiant disorder
Conduct disorder
Internalizing disorders
Eating disorders
Anorexia nervosa
Bulimia nervosa
Developmental psychopathology
Developmental norms
Life span development
Externalizing symptoms
Syndrome
Symptom
Socialization
Self-control
Adolescent-limited
Life-course-persistent
Cognitive capacity
Separation anxiety disorder
Peer sociometric method
Reactivity
Adultomorphism
Isomorphic
Pica
Rumination disorder
Tourette's disorder
Selective mutism
Reactive attachment disorder
Stereotypic movement disorder
Encopresis
Enuresis
Learning disabilities/speech and hearing problems
Academic aptitude
Academic achievement tests
Minimal brain damage (MBD)
Psychostimulants
Juvenile delinquency

Status offenses
Criminal offenses
Sustained attention
Representative sample
Generalize
Population of interest
Testosterone
Cluster suicides
Family adversity index
Anxious attachment
Resilience
Coercion
Time-out
Negative attention
Delay of gratification
Soft signs
"Feingold diet"
Salicylates
Socialized delinquency
Dose-response effects
Behavioral family therapy
Negotiation
Achievement place
Recidivism
Rehabilitation
Parens patriae
Diversion
Distorted body image
Hypothalamus
Structural family therapy

KEY NAMES

The following individuals have made important contributions to the material presented in the chapter. Write out the names of these individuals and the theories, research, or treatment with which they are associated. Then check your answers with the information in your text.

Mary Ainsworth
George Still
Lightner Witmer
Charles Bradley
Nicholas Zill

Michael Rutter
John Bowlby
Lawrence Kohlberg
Sir William Withey Gull

MATCHING QUESTIONS

Match the following terms and names with the definitions presented below. The answers can be found at the end of the chapter.

a. externalizing symptoms
b. adultomorphism
c. pica
d. anorexia nervosa
e. reactive attachment disorder
f. rumination disorder
g. reactivity
h. Lightner Witmer
i. separation anxiety
j. bulimia nervosa

k. George Still
l. juvenile delinquency
m. authoritarian
n. time-out
o. learning disabilities
p. negotiation
q. conduct disorder
r. status offenses
s. diversion
t. authoritative

1) _____ a disorder characterized by drastically restricted eating and extreme emaciation

2) _____ the persistent eating of nonnutritive substances such as paint or dirt

3) _____ type of parenting style in which parents are both loving and firm in disciplining their children

4) _____ a disorder characterized by severely disturbed and developmentally inappropriate social relationships

5) _____ the subclassification of externalizing disorders can be traced to this man, who wrote about the condition that we know today as attention-deficit/hyperactivity disorder

6) _____ a normal fear that typically develops in the months just before a baby's first birthday

7) _____ the goal of this "treatment" is to keep problem youth out of the juvenile justice system

8) _____ this is a legal classification, not a mental disorder

9) _____ the repeat offending of a delinquent behavior following treatment

10) _____ characterized by violations of age-appropriate social rules such as disobedience, aggression, and perhaps legal violations

11) _____ the individual who established the first psychological clinic for children in the United States at the University of Pennsylvania

12) _____ central to behavior family therapy with adolescents, this is a process in which young people are actively involved in defining rules

13) _____ type of parenting style in which the parents lack warmth, and discipline is strict and often harsh and undemocratic

14) _____ a disorder distinguished by frequent episodes of binge eating followed by intentional purging

15) _____ technique of briefly isolating a child following misbehavior

16) _____ the belief that children suffer from the same psychological disorders as adults

17) _____ this disorder is defined primarily by forms of behavior such as stealing or assault that are illegal as well as antisocial

18) _____ a heterogeneous group of problems that are characterized by a difference between academic aptitude and academic performance

19) _____ primarily found among infants, this is the repeated regurgitation and rechewing of food

20) _____ changes in behavior that occur simply as a result of being observed

MULTIPLE CHOICE QUESTIONS

The following multiple choice questions will test your comprehension of the material presented in the chapter. Circle the correct choice for each question in the section. Then compare your answers with those at the end of the chapter.

1) All of the following are major problems in evaluating children's internalizing symptoms EXCEPT:

a. there are insufficient self-report measures to assess internalizing symptoms in children

b. it is much more difficult for adults to assess children's inner experiences than it is to observe children's behavior

c. children often are not reliable or valid informants about their internal life

d. children's capacity to recognize emotions in themselves emerges slowly over the course of development and therefore they may not be aware of their own emotional turmoil

2) In his study on family adversity, Michael Rutter found that all of the following were predictors of behavior problems among children EXCEPT:

a. low income
b. overcrowding in the home
c. conflict between parents
d. paternal depression

3) Reactive attachment disorder is most likely caused by which of the following?

a. it appears to have genetic origins
b. an unstable home environment in which care providers are frequently changing
c. extremely neglectful parenting
d. its etiology is unknown

4) Both bulimia and anorexia nervosa are characterized by which of the following?

a. struggle for control
b. considerable shame
c. obsessive-compulsive disorder
d. the absence of menstruation

5) All of the following are major subtypes of externalizing disorders EXCEPT:

a. attention-deficit/hyperactivity disorder
b. conduct disorder
c. depression
d. oppositional defiant disorder

6) Which of the following is the most helpful information for scientists to have for predicting adult antisocial behavior?

a. information obtained during birth and infancy
b. information obtained during childhood

c. information obtained during adolescence

d. information obtained during adulthood

7) According to a panel of experts assembled by the National Academy of Sciences, at least _____ percent of the 63 million children living in the United States suffer from a mental disorder:

    a. 5

    b. 12

    c. 17

    d. 23

8) Which of the following is a sample that accurately depicts some larger group of people?

    a. representative sample

    b. random sample

    c. convenience sample

    d. heterogeneous sample

9) _____ implies that an externalizing problem has environmental origins, while _____ implies problems with some sort of biological cause.

    a. attention-deficit/hyperactivity disorder; oppositional defiant disorder

    b. oppositional defiant disorder; attention-deficit/hyperactivity disorder

    c. conduct disorder; oppositional defiant disorder

    d. oppositional defiant disorder; conduct disorder

10) Separation anxiety disorder is typically associated with all of the following EXCEPT:

    a. fears of getting lost or being kidnapped

    b. refusal to be alone

    c. persistent and excessive worry for the safety of an attachment figure

    d. refusal to interact with others when the attachment figure is not present

11) Typically, the attachment figure for an infant with an anxious attachment responds to the infant in which of the following ways?

    a. appropriately attends to the infant's needs

    b. inadequately or inconsistently attends to the infant's needs

    c. immediately attends to the infant's needs

    d. is completely unresponsive to the infant's needs

12) The FBI reports that approximately _____ percent of arrests for major crimes including murder, forcible rape, and robbery are of juveniles under the age of 18.

a. 10
b. 20
c. 30
d. 40

13) Which of the following is a well-known treatment device that awakens children with enuresis by setting off an alarm as they begin to wet the bed during the night?

a. bell and pad
b. light and alarm
c. sensitive signal seat
d. responsive wetting device

14) All of the following are compensatory behaviors of bulimia nervosa EXCEPT:

a. misuse of laxatives
b. complete avoidance of food
c. intense exercise
d. misuse of enemas

15) All of the following are symptoms of anorexia nervosa EXCEPT:

a. an intense fear of gaining weight
b. refusal to maintain weight at or above minimally normal weight for age and height
c. acknowledgement of the seriousness of low body weight, but refusal to change eating behavior
d. amenorrhea, or the absence of menstruation

16) Which of the following is characterized by self-stimulation or self-injurious behavior?

a. conduct disorder
b. developmental coordination disorder
c. Tourette's disorder
d. stereotypic movement disorder

17) Treatment with children often begins with which of the following?

a. an attempt to get the adults (i.e., parents, teachers) to agree as to what the problem really is
b. identifying a disorder and then building hypotheses to either prove or disprove it
c. helping the child to identify his or her problems
d. an attempt to treat the family, independent of the child, in order to facilitate change in the child's environment

18) Attention-deficit/hyperactivity disorder is characterized by all of the following symptoms EXCEPT:

    a. impulsivity
    b. hyperactivity
    c. aggression
    d. inattention

19) Which of the following theories offers the most promising explanations for eating disorders?

    a. biological
    b. social
    c. psychological
    d. all of the above equally offer promising explanations of eating disorders

20) Which of the following gender differences is NOT TRUE in respect to internalizing and externalizing problems?

    a. more adult men enter into therapy than do adult women
    b. boys are treated more for psychological problems than are girls
    c. by early adult life, more females report psychological problems than males
    d. boys have far more externalizing disorders than girls

21) According to the "peer sociometric method" of assessing children's relationships, which of the following groups is characterized by a high frequency of "liked least" ratings and a low frequency of "liked most" ratings?

    a. average
    b. neglected
    c. rejected
    d. controversial

22) All of the following are symptoms of bulimia nervosa EXCEPT:

    a. recurrent episodes of binge eating that involve large amounts of food
    b. occurs solely during episodes of anorexia nervosa
    c. recurrent inappropriate compensatory behavior, especially purging
    d. undue influence of weight and body shape on self-evaluation

23) Both bulimia and anorexia nervosa are approximately _____ times more common among women than among men.

a. 10
b. 15
c. 20
d. 25

24) All of the following are internalizing symptoms EXCEPT:

a. somatic complaints
b. fears
c. aggressive behavior
d. sadness

25) Many professionals agree that anorexia is a source of which of the following?

a. shame
b. pride
c. gratification
d. resentment

26) All of the following factors influence how adults evaluate children's rule violations EXCEPT:

a. frequency of the child's behavior
b. duration of the child's behavior
c. intensity of the child's behavior
d. all of the above

27) Brandon is a 3-year-old who frequently throws a tantrum when in the grocery store if he does not get what he wants. Because this is such an embarrassing situation for his mother, she will give Brandon whatever he desires in order to get his cooperation. In this case, Brandon is being _____ while his mother is being _____.

a. positively reinforced; negatively reinforced
b. negatively reinforced; positively reinforced
c. classically conditioned; punished
d. positively reinforced; punished

28) Minimal brain damage (MBD) is a hypothesis that has been used to explain which disorder?

a. oppositional defiant disorder
b. conduct disorder
c. attention-deficit/hyperactivity disorder
d. Tourette's disorder

29) Infants typically develop a fear of _____ around the age of 7 to 8 months.

    a. strangers
    b. the dark
    c. monsters
    d. unfamiliar environments

30) Which of the following is the process of shaping children's behavior and attitudes to conform to the expectations of parents, teachers, and society as a whole?

    a. modeling
    b. socialization
    c. conditioning
    d. vicarious learning

BRIEF ESSAY

As a final exercise, write out answers to the following brief essay questions. Then compare your answers with the material presented in the text.

After you have answered these questions, review the "Critical Thinking" questions that are presented at the end of the text chapter. Answering these questions will help you integrate important issues and themes that have been featured throughout the chapter.

1. Briefly describe the study conducted by Lobitz and Johnson. What do their findings suggest? What must we be cautious of in interpreting the results?

2. Your text discusses classifying children's psychological problems in the context of key interpersonal relationships rather than using the current method of classification. Briefly discuss the strengths and weaknesses of each approach.

3. Compare and contrast the following disorders: attention-deficit/hyperactivity disorder, oppositional defiant disorder, and conduct disorder. Include a brief discussion on the overlap between these disorders.

4. If you were a therapist and a young woman entered therapy for an eating disorder, what would your treatment plan entail? Would your treatment for a male patient differ from treatment for a female patient? Explain why or why not.

ANSWER KEY

MATCHING EXERCISES

1. d	11. h
2. c	12. p
3. t	13. m
4. e	14. j
5. k	15. n
6. i	16. b
7. s	17. q
8. l	18. o
9. r	19. f
10. a	20. g

MULTIPLE CHOICE EXERCISES

1. a	6. b	11. b
2. d	7. b	12. c
3. c	8. a	13. a
4. a	9. b	14. b
5. c	10. d	15. c

16. d	21. c	26. d
17. a	22. b	27. a
18. c	23. a	28. c
19. b	24. c	29. a
20. a	25. b	30. b

CHAPTER SIXTEEN
LIFE CYCLE TRANSITIONS AND ADULT DEVELOPMENT

CHAPTER OUTLINE

Overview
    Typical Symptoms and Associated Features
    Classifications of Life Cycle Transitions
        Brief Historical Perspective
        Contemporary Views of Life Cycle Transitions

The Transition to Adulthood
    Typical Symptoms and Associated Features
        Identity Crisis
        Changes in Roles and Relationships
        Emotional Turmoil
    Classification of Identity Conflicts
    Epidemiology of Identity Conflicts
    Etiological Considerations and Research
    Treatment During the Transition to Adult Life

Family Transitions
    Typical Symptoms and Associated Features
        Family Conflict
        Emotional Distress
        Cognitive Conflicts
    Classification of Family Relationships
    Epidemiology of Family Transitions
    Etiological Considerations and Research
        Psychological Factors
            Communication Problems
            Family Roles
        Social Factors
        Biological Factors
    Treatment During Family Transitions
        Prevention Programs
        Marital and Family Therapy
            Behavioral Marital Therapy
            Treating Individual Problems with Marital and Family Therapy

Aging and the Transition to Later Life
    Typical Symptoms and Associated Features
        Grief and Bereavement

LEARNING OBJECTIVES

After reviewing the material presented in this chapter, you should be able to:

* define life-cycle transition

* understand that life-cycle transitions may play a role in the development of psychopathology

* describe Erikson's psychosocial moratorium and identity crisis

* define Marcia's four identity statuses

* describe some common gender differences which occur in the transition to adulthood

* identify ways in which power struggles, intimacy struggles, affiliation, interdependence, and scapegoating impact upon the family structure

* describe Gottman's four communication problems, giving examples for each type of problem

* describe some premarital and marital therapy treatment programs

* compare Bowlby's and Kubler-Ross's model of grieving in bereavement

* identify typical psychological and physiological processes in young-old, old-old, and oldest-old adults

* describe some gender differences in adults in later life in terms of relationships

KEY TERMS AND CONCEPTS

Following is a list of key terms and concepts that are featured in the chapter and are important for you to know. Write out the definitions of each of these terms and check your answers with the definitions in the text.

Life cycle transitions
Transition to adult life
Family transitions
Transition to later life
Developmental tasks of adult life
Interpersonal diagnoses
Crisis of the healthy personality
Grief
Identity
"V codes"
Identity versus role confusion
Identity crisis
Intimacy versus self-absorption
Generactivity versus stagnation
Integrity and despair
Family life cycle
Early adult transition
Midlife transition
Late adult transition
Moratorium
Identity diffusion
Identity foreclosure
Identity moratorium
Identity achievement
Alienated identity achievement
"Forgotten half"
Empty nest
Power struggles
Intimacy struggles
Boundaries
Reciprocity
Affiliation
Interdependence
Scapegoat
Heritability

Heritability ratio
Criticism
Contempt
Defensiveness
Stonewalling
Marital and family therapy
Behavioral marital therapy
Menopause
Estrogen
Hormone replacement therapy
Bereavement
Reminiscence
Integrative reminiscence
Instrumental reminiscence
Transitive reminiscence
Escapist reminiscence
Obsessive reminiscence
Narrative reminiscence
Integrative reminiscence
Gerontology
Young-old adults
Old-old adults
Oldest-old adults
Behavioral gerontology

KEY NAMES

The following individuals have made important contributions to the material presented in the chapter. Write out the names of these individuals and the theories, research, or treatment with which they are associated. Then check your answers with the information in your text.

Erik Erikson
Daniel Levinson
Karen Horney
Lorna Benjamin
John Gottman
Matt McGue
David Lykken
Elisabeth Kubler-Ross
Paul Wong
Lisa Watt

MATCHING QUESTIONS

Match the following terms and names with the definitions presented below. The answers can be found at the end of the chapter.

a. identity
b. scapegoat
c. interpersonal diagnosis
d. identity diffusion
e. grief
f. contempt
g. reciprocity
h. empty nest
i. identity foreclosure
j. developmental tasks of adult life

k. escapist reminiscence
l. early adult transition
m. ageism
n. behavioral gerontology
o. identity crisis
p. marital and family therapy
q. menopause
r. defensiveness
s. gerontology
t. obsessive reminiscence

1) _____ the process of never questioning oneself or one's goals but instead preceding along the predetermined course of one's childhood commitments

2) _____ includes glorifying one's past life and depreciating one's present life (e.g., a yearning for the "good old days")

3) _____ a period of basic uncertainty about oneself

4) _____ fairly predictable challenges in work, life goals, relationships, and personal identity that occur during the course of the adult years

5) _____ according to Levinson, this stage involves moving away from family and assuming adult roles

6) _____ a family member who is held to blame for all of the family's troubles

7) _____ the social exchange of cooperation and conflict in family interactions

8) _____ a form of social prejudice that encompasses a number of misconceptions and biases about aging

9) _____ an insult that may be motivated by anger and is intended to hurt the other person

10) _____ the emotional and social process of coping with a separation or loss

11) _____ the cessation of menstruation in older women

12) _____   one's global sense of self

13) _____   a discipline developed specifically for studying and diagnosing the behavioral components of health and illness among older adults

14) _____   the process of questioning one's childhood identity but not actively searching for new adult roles

15) _____   a recollection of one's past which includes a preoccupation with failure and is full of guilt, bitterness, and despair

16) _____   a system of conceptualizing psychological problems as residing within the context of relationships and not just within the individual

17) _____   an approach that focuses on changing relationships, rather than on changing the individual

18) _____   a form of self-justification such as denying responsibility or blaming another person

19) _____   the adjustment that occurs when adult children leave the family home

20) _____   the multidisciplinary study of aging

MULTIPLE CHOICE QUESTIONS

The following multiple choice questions will test your comprehension of the material presented in the chapter. Circle the correct choice for each question in the section. Then compare your answers with those at the end of the chapter.

1) According to Lorna Benjamin, the foundation of this dimension of relationships is attack at one end and active love at the opposite extreme.

     a. interdependence
     b. enmeshed
     c. affiliation
     d. resolution

2) Which of the following groups has the highest suicide rate?

     a. teenagers
     b. young adults

c. middle-aged adults

d. adults over the age of 65

3) Which of the following includes various struggles in the process of moving from one social or psychological "stage" of adult development into a new stage?

    a. life cycle transitions
    b. transition to adult life
    c. developmental tasks of adult life
    d. family transitions

4) Approximately _____ of couples seen in behavioral marital therapy do not improve significantly.

    a. 30%
    b. 40%
    c. 50%
    d. 60%

5) According to Erikson, which of the following stages is the major challenge of adolescence and young adulthood?

    a. integrity versus despair
    b. generativity versus stagnation
    c. intimacy versus self-absorption
    d. identity versus role confusion

6) On the average, marital happiness declines following _____.

    a. the death of a family member
    b. the birth of the first child
    c. the emptying of the family nest
    d. the fifth year of marriage

7) Which of the following refers to youth who do not attend college and who often assume marginal roles in U.S. society?

    a. "Transient Youth"
    b. "Generation X"
    c. "Alienated Youth"
    d. "Forgotten Half"

8) Research indicates that depression is more closely linked to _____ for women, while it is more closely liked to _____ for men.

a. marital conflict; divorce

b. divorce; marital conflict

c. poor support system; financial difficulties

d. financial difficulties; poor support system

9) When reviewing the various models of adult development, which of the following must be taken into consideration?

a. that history, culture, and personal values influence views about which kinds of "tasks" are normal during adult development

b. that transitions or "crises" may not be as predictable as the models imply

c. some people may not pass through a particular stage of development

d. all of the above

10) The ratio of men to women _____ at older ages.

a. increases

b. decreases

c. is approximately equal

d. stays relatively the same across the age span

11) Erik Erikson highlighted _____ as a common theme that occurs throughout life cycle transitions.

a. uncertainty

b. conflict

c. remorse

d. acceptance

12) Estimates indicate that about _____ of all of today's marriages will end in divorce.

a. 30%

b. 40%

c. 50%

d. 60%

13) Epidemiological evidence indicates that the prevalence of mental disorders is _____ among adults 65 years of age and older as compared to younger adults.

a. lower

b. higher

c. about the same

d. it is unknown due to the difficulty in studying this population

14) Which of the following identifies people who are in the middle of an identity crisis and who are actively searching for adult roles?

    a. alienated identity achievement
    b. identity moratorium
    c. identify diffusion
    d. identity foreclosure

15) All of the following are emphasized by behavioral marital therapy EXCEPT:

    a. the couple's moment-to-moment interactions
    b. strategies for solving problems
    c. extensive clinical interview of relationship patterns in the couple's families
    d. the couple's style of communication

16) Family life cycle theorists classify adult development according to which of the following?

    a. the tasks and transitions of family life
    b. the adult's memories of their childhood and adolescence
    c. the tasks and transitions of psychological challenges of adulthood
    d. all of the above

17) Psychological research suggests that the most successful young adults have which kind of parents?

    a. parents who are strict and authoritarian
    b. parents who are supportive and could be characterized as their children's "best friend"
    c. parents who strongly encourage individuation and provide opportunities for their children to take on numerous responsibilities at an early age
    d. parents who strike a balance between continuing to provide support and supervision of their children while allowing them increasing independence

18) Which of the following individuals theorized that people have competing needs to move toward, to move away from, and to move against others?

    a. Erik Erikson
    b. Daniel Levinson
    c. Karen Horney
    d. Elisabeth Kubler-Ross

19) _____ struggles are attempts to change dominance relations, whereas _____ struggles are attempts to alter the degree of closeness in a relationship.

    a. intimacy; power
    b. power; intimacy
    c. conflict; relational
    d. relational; conflict

20) A study of adults over the age of 70 found that both men and women listed which of the following as the most common contribution to a negative quality of life in their later years?

    a. poor health
    b. death of a spouse
    c. financial difficulties
    d. interpersonal problems

21) All of the following are true of the "V codes" in the DSM-IV EXCEPT:

    a. they do not include an extensive summary of life difficulties
    b. they are similar to other diagnoses in the DSM in that they are diagnosed as mental disorders
    c. they include issues such as bereavement, identity problems, and phase of life problems.
    d. all of the above are true of "V codes"

22) Lisa and Mike have been married for four years. Recently, they have been arguing more than usual. Whenever they get into an argument, Lisa engages in a pattern of isolation and withdrawal, ignoring Mike's complaints and virtually ceasing all communication with him. According to the four basic communication problems identified by John Gottman, Lisa is engaged in which of the following?:

    a. stonewalling
    b. contempt
    c. defensiveness
    d. criticism

23) According to your text, all of the following are true of hormone replacement therapy EXCEPT:

    a. it alleviates some of the psychological strains associated with adverse physical symptoms of menopause
    b. reduces the subsequent risk for heart and bone disease
    c. increases the risk for cancer

d. decreases symptoms of depression, which are often associated with menopause

24) Alternative lifestyles not withstanding, evidence indicates that _____ of the adults in the United States get married during their adult lives.

a. 40%
b. 60%
c. 75%
d. 90%

25) One criticism of Erikson's theories is:

a. the stages are inappropriate for certain developmental levels
b. the theories are too broad and general and are not applicable to a large proportion of the population
c. they are not very accurate in outlining developmental stages
d. the theories focus on men to the exclusion of women

26) According to Canadian psychologists Paul Wong and Lisa Watt, which of the following is associated with less successful adjustment in later life?

a. obsessive reminiscence
b. transitive reminiscence
c. instrumental reminiscence
d. integrative reminiscence

27) Family therapists and family researchers often blame difficulties in negotiating family transitions on which of the following?

a. low motivation
b. problems with communication
c. difficulty identifying problem areas
d. all of the above

28) Which of the following is NOT a stage of adult development in Erikson's model?

a. intimacy versus self-absorption
b. integrity versus despair
c. assurance versus apprehension
d. generativity versus stagnation

29) Research on identity achievement indicates that _____ may have rejecting and distant families, while _____ may have overprotective families.

a. identity diffusers; identity foreclosers
b. identity foreclosers; identity diffusers
c. identity achievers; alienated identity achievers
d. alienated identity achievers; identity achievers

30) All of the following are stages included in the Family Developmental Tasks through the Family Life Cycle EXCEPT:

a. childbearing
b. launching center
c. aging family members
d. death and dying

BRIEF ESSAY

As a final exercise, write out answers to the following brief essay questions. Then compare your answers with the material presented in the text.

After you have answered these questions, review the "Critical Thinking" questions that are presented at the end of the text chapter. Answering these questions will help you integrate important issues and themes that have been featured throughout the chapter.

1. Discuss the stages of Erik Erikson's model of adult development. What do you consider to be the strengths of this model? What are some of its weaknesses?

2. Outline the psychological, social, and biological factors that may contribute to difficulties in family transitions. Which factors do you think are most important when identifying the etiology of family transition difficulties?

3. Review the six categories of reminiscence identified by Paul Wong and Lisa Watt. Which categories appear to be related to successful aging? Which appear to be associated with less successful adjustment in later life? Which category do you think will best describe your reminiscence later in life? Why?

4. Discuss the various categories of identity conflicts as presented in your text. Presently, which category do you fit best in? Why?

ANSWER KEY

MATCHING EXERCISES

1. i	11. q
2. k	12. a
3. o	13. n
4. j	14. d
5. l	15. t
6. b	16. c
7. g	17. p
8. m	18. r
9. f	19. h
10. e	20. s

MULTIPLE CHOICE EXERCISES

1. c	6. b	11. b
2. d	7. d	12. c
3. a	8. a	13. a
4. c	9. d	14. b
5. d	10. b	15. c
16. a	21. b	26. a
17. d	22. a	27. b
18. c	23. d	28. c
19. b	24. d	29. a
20. a	25. d	30. d

CHAPTER SEVENTEEN
MENTAL HEALTH AND THE LAW

CHAPTER OUTLINE

LEARNING OBJECTIVES

After reviewing the material presented in this chapter, you should be able to:

*   understand the "free will vs. determinism" issue and its role in the insanity defense

*   distinguish the M'Naghten test, the irresistible impulse test, the product test, and the American Law Institute model legislation for determining insanity

*   describe the "guilty but mentally ill" verdict and explain the consequences of such a verdict

*   know the basic statistics surrounding the use of the "not guilty by reason of insanity" (NGRI) plea and compare the consequences given the verdict of NGRI with that of a "guilty" verdict

*   understand the issue of "competence" and the role it plays in the legal system

*   contrast the libertarian position with that of the paternalist position regarding involuntary psychiatric commitment to an inpatient hospital

*   understand the reasons for the unreliability of dangerous predictions and suicide risk predictions

*   describe the basic issues involved in the psychiatric patient's right to treatment, the right to the least restrictive alternative environment, and the right to refuse treatment

*   understand some of the problems associated with the deinstitutionalization movement in psychiatry

*   describe the role of mental health practitioners in child custody disputes

*   delineate some of the most common types of malpractice cases that are filed against mental health practitioners

*   list some situations in which psychologists are legally bound to break confidentiality

KEY TERMS AND CONCEPTS

Following is a list of key terms and concepts that are featured in the chapter and are important for you to know. Write out the definitions of each of these terms and check your answers with the definitions in the text.

Insanity defense
Free will
Criminal responsibility
Determinism
M'Naghten test
Irresistible impulse test
Deterrence
Product test
Guilty but mentally ill (GBMI)
Burden of proof
Standard of proof
Competence
Miranda warning
Moral treatment
Libertarian
Paternalist
Preventive detention
Civil commitment
Parens patriae
Police power
Emergency commitment procedures
Formal commitment procedures
Base rates
Right to treatment
Right to refuse treatment

Informed consent
Substituted judgment
Deinstitutionalization
Revolving door phenomenon
Family law
Child custody
Physical custody
Legal custody
Joint custody
Child's best interests standard
Mediators
Battered woman syndrome
"Cycle of violence"
Child abuse
Physical child abuse
Child sexual abuse
Child neglect
Psychological abuse
Foster care
Professional responsibilities
Negligence
Malpractice
Confidentiality
Privileged communications

KEY NAMES

The following individuals/cases have made important contributions to the material presented in the chapter. Write out the names of these individuals or the court cases presented and the theories, research, or treatment with which they are associated. Then check your answers with the information in your text.

Thomas Szasz
Parsons v. State
Durham v. United States
Benjamin Rush
Phillipe Pinel
William Tuke
Dorothea Dix
Mrs. E.P.W. Packard
John Monahan
Parham v. J.R.
Lois Weithorn
Wyatt v. Stickney

O'Connor v. Donaldson
Lake v. Cameron
Washington v. Harper
Bertram Brown
E. Fuller Torrey
Lenore Walker
Henry Kempe
Osheroff v. Chestnut Lodge
Tarasoff v. Regents of the University of California

MATCHING QUESTIONS

Match the following terms and names with the definitions presented below. The answers can be found at the end of the chapter.

a. irresistible impulse test
b. civil commitment
c. free will
d. moral treatment
e. paternalist view
f. M'Naghten test
g. revolving door
h. competence
i. psychological abuse
j. determinism

k. parens patriae
l. mediators
m. foster care
n. preventive detention
o. negligence
p. child's best interests standard
q. malpractice
r. child neglect
s. libertarian view
t. deinstitutionalization

1) _____ this movement led to improved conditions in some mental hospitals

2) _____ this is the involuntary hospitalization of the mentally ill

3) _____ this involves placing a child at risk for serious physical or psychological harm by failing to provide basic and expected care

4) _____ the capacity to make choices and freely act upon them

5) _____ a law that governs custody disputes

6) _____ this refers to situations in which professional negligence results in harm to clients or patients

7) _____ this indicated that defendants could be found insane if they were unable to control their actions because of mental disease

8) _____   this emphasizes the state's duty to protect its citizens

9) _____   this occurs when a professional fails to perform in a manner that is consistent with the level of skill exercised by other professionals in the field

10) _____   the philosophy that the government has a humanitarian responsibility to care for its weaker members

11) _____   this is confinement before a crime is actually committed

12) _____   this refers to the phenomenon in which more patients are admitted to psychiatric hospitals more frequently but for shorter periods of time

13) _____   a program designed primarily to help children who are in physical danger

14) _____   the assumption that human behavior results from biological, psychological, and social forces

15) _____   professionals who meet with divorcing parents and help them to identify, negotiate, and ultimately resolve their disputes

16) _____   the philosophy that many of the mentally ill and mentally retarded can be better cared for in their community than in large mental hospitals

17) _____   this refers to repeated denigration in the absence of physical harm

18) _____   this concerns the defendants' ability to understand the legal proceedings that are taking place against them and to participate in their own defense

19) _____   this emphasizes protecting the rights of the individual

20) _____   this clearly explained the "right from wrong" principle for determining insanity

MULTIPLE CHOICE QUESTIONS

The following multiple choice questions will test your comprehension of the material presented in the chapter. Circle the correct choice for each question in the section. Then compare your answers with those at the end of the chapter.

1) Which of the following cases ruled that a state could not confine a non-dangerous individual who is capable of surviving safely on their own or with the help of willing and responsible family members or friends?

    a. Washington v. Harper
    b. Parham v. J.R.
    c. O'Connor v. Donaldson
    d. Lake v. Cameron

2) _____ commitment procedures allow an acutely disturbed individual to be temporarily confined in a mental hospital, typically for no more than a few days, while _____ commitment procedures can lead to involuntary hospitalization that is ordered by the court and typically lasts for much longer.

    a. formal; emergency
    b. emergency; formal
    c. medical; crisis
    d. crisis; medical

3) All of the following are true of the "guilty but mentally ill" (GBMI) verdict EXCEPT:

    a. holds defendants criminally responsible for their crimes
    b. helps ensure that the defendant receives treatment for the mental disorder
    c. it was designed as a compromise to the "not guilty by reason of insanity" (NGRI) verdict
    d. a defendant found to be GBMI cannot be sentenced in the same manner as any criminal

4) All of the following have been goals of deinstitutionalization EXCEPT:

    a. to prevent inappropriate mental hospital admissions through arranging community alternatives to treatment
    b. to release to the community all institutionalized patients who have been given adequate preparation for such a change
    c. to decrease the influx of mental health patients by not allowing them continued access to mental hospitals and thus encouraging independence
    d. to establish and maintain community support systems for non-institutionalized people receiving mental health services in the community

5) Which of the following individuals argues that mental disorders are subjective "problems in living" rather than objective diseases, and thus believes that the concept of mental illness is a myth?

    a. Thomas Szasz
    b. E. Fuller Torrey
    c. Bertram Brown
    d. Henry Kempe

6) The majority of custody decisions are made by:

    a. parents themselves
    b. attorneys who negotiate for the parents outside of court
    c. a judge and decided in court
    d. mental health professionals who evaluate the case

7) All of the following are true of the parens patriae EXCEPT:

    a. it is used to justify the state's supervision of minors and
       incapacitated adults
    b. it is based on the state's duty to protect the public safety, health,
       and welfare
    c. commitment under these rationales was virtually unknown to the United
       States until the early 1950's
    d. it refers to the concept of the "state as parent"

8) Following a civil commitment to a mental hospital, mental patients' rights include all of the following EXCEPT:

    a. right to treatment
    b. right to design their own treatment plan
    c. right to refuse treatment
    d. right to treatment in the least restrictive alternative environment

9) Evidence suggests that the insanity defense is used in approximately _____ of all criminal cases in the United States.

    a. 1%
    b. 4%
    c. 7%
    d. 10%

10) All of the following stages are part of Lenore Walker's stages of the "cycle of violence" EXCEPT:

a. battering incident
b. tension-building phase
c. loving contrition
d. verbal reprimands

11) On the average, defendants who are found "not guilty by reason of insanity" (NGRI) spend _____ time confined in an institution as they would have if they had been given a prison sentence instead.

a. significantly less
b. twice as much
c. approximately the same
d. roughly three times as much

12) Which of the following terms is defined as the ethical obligation not to reveal private communication and is basic to psychotherapy?

a. confidentiality
b. private communications
c. classified information
d. privileged communications

13) Mental disorders and the actions that result from them are typically viewed as:

a. choices
b. conditions that are outside of voluntary control
c. responsibilities that the mentally disordered individual must assume
d. a and c

14) All of the following are issues of special relevance regarding involuntary hospitalization of the severely mentally impaired EXCEPT:

a. criminal record
b. civil commitment
c. patients' rights
d. deinstitutionalization

15) The acquittal of John Hinckley prompted all of the following EXCEPT:

a. the new verdict "guilty but mentally ill" (GBMI)
b. a revised definition of the insanity defense
c. shifting the burden of proof from the prosecution to the defense in federal courts

d. the creation of a much stricter standard of proof for the defense in the majority of states

16) Research indicates that approximately _____ of the mentally disturbed are not violent.

    a. 30%
    b. 50%
    c. 70%
    d. 90%

17) All of the following are grounds that tend to dominate commitment laws EXCEPT:

    a. being dangerous to others
    b. inability to care for self
    c. being dangerous to self
    d. inability to care for others

18) Over _____ of all reports of child abuse are found to be unsubstantiated after an investigation.

    a. one-eighth
    b. one-quarter
    c. one-half
    d. two-thirds

19) All of the following were key figures in instituting moral treatment reform efforts for the mentally ill EXCEPT:

    a. Benjamin Rush
    b. Lenore Walker
    c. Phillipe Pinel
    d. Dorothea Dix

20) Empirical research on the adjustment of children from divorced families indicates that:

    a. a substantial portion of the difficulties found among children after divorce actually begins long before the marital separation occurs
    b. the psychological functioning of children from divorced families does not differ from that of children from non-divorced families
    c. the difficulties children experience are directly related to marital conflict and divorce
    d. children from divorced families tend to have more internalizing problems than children from non-divorced families

21) Which of the following is known as the "product test" and indicated that "an accused is not criminally responsible if his unlawful act was the product of mental disease or defect"?

    a. Parsons v. State
    b. O'Connor v. Donaldson
    c. Durham v. United States
    d. Parham v. J.R.

22) One of the more common malpractice claims against mental health professionals is:

    a. the misuse of psychotherapeutic techniques
    b. the inappropriate use of electroconvulsive therapy (ECT)
    c. the failure to disclose therapeutic interpretations to clients
    d. inappropriate hospitalization

23) Confidentiality between a therapist and a client can be broken under which of the following circumstances?

    a. the client is threatening to harm another person
    b. the client has disclosed sexual or physical abuse of a child
    c. the client is threatening to harm himself or herself
    d. all of the above

24) Which of the following is NOT TRUE of the legal definition of "competence"?

    a. it refers to the defendant's ability to understand criminal proceedings
    b. it refers to the defendant's current mental status
    c. it refers to the defendants willingness to participate in criminal
       proceedings
    d. the "reasonable degree" of understanding needed to establish competence
       is generally acknowledged to be fairly low

25) In the case of Wyatt v. Stickney, the federal district court ruled that at a minimum, public mental institutions must provide all of the following EXCEPT:

    a. a humane psychological and physical environment
    b. a sufficient number of qualified staff to administer adequate treatment
    c. individualized treatment plans
    d. "reasonable" rates for inpatient services

26) Which of the following details a suspect's rights to remain silent and to have an attorney present during police questioning?

a. Miranda warning
b. informed consent
c. confidentiality
d. parens patriae

27) Evidence suggests that in child custody cases, mediation:

a. does not necessarily reduce the number of custody hearings in court
b. is more effective than the role that mental health professionals play
   in custody cases, and thus mental health professionals should limit
   their involvement in the legal system
c. does not help parents reach decisions more quickly than if they were to
   go through custody hearings in court
d. is viewed by parents as more favorable than litigation, especially fathers

28) Which of the following cases established the patient's right to be treated in the least restrictive alternative environment?

a. Lake v. Cameron
b. Osheroff v. Chestnut Lodge
c. O'Connor v. Donaldson
d. none of the above

29) Which of the following is TRUE regarding the idea that mental disability should limit criminal responsibility?

a. it is a relatively new concept among mental health professionals
b. it dates back to ancient Greek and Hebrew traditions and was evident in
   early English law
c. it has emerged in our legal system within the past 50 years
d. it surfaced following World War II when large numbers of veterans who
   experienced post-traumatic stress symptoms and committed violent acts

30) In his research on the prediction of dangerousness, John Monahon has found which of the following to be several times higher among prison inmates as among the general population?

a. major depression
b. bipolar disorder
c. schizophrenia
d. all of the above

BRIEF ESSAY

As a final exercise, write out answers to the following brief essay questions. Then compare your answers with the material presented in the text.

After you have answered these questions, review the "Critical Thinking" questions that are presented at the end of the text chapter. Answering these questions will help you integrate important issues and themes that have been featured throughout the chapter.

1. Joe is a 35 year-old white male who was recently arrested for sexually abusing a seven year-old girl. Although this is Joe's first offense, he has a history of "sexual addictions" that range from viewing pornography while masturbating to exhibitionism. Explain how you think criminal law would conceptualize Joe's behavior and how you think a mental health professional would conceptualize Joe's behavior. Discuss the similarities and differences of the two conceptualizations.

2. Briefly discuss Thomas Szasz's position on free will and determinism, mental illness, and the insanity defense. Do you agree or disagree with Szasz? Why?

3. What are the basic underlying principles of libertarianism and paternalism? Which view do you most agree with? Defend your position.

4. Discuss the implications of the Tarasoff v. Regents of the University of California case. If you would have been the therapist of Prosenjit Poddar, would you have handled the situation differently? Why or why not?

ANSWER KEY

MATCHING EXERCISES

1. d	11. n
2. b	12. g
3. r	13. m
4. c	14. j
5. p	15. l
6. q	16. t
7. a	17. i
8. e	18. h
9. o	19. s
10. k	20. f

MULTIPLE CHOICE EXERCISES

1. c	6. b	11. c
2. b	7. c	12. a
3. d	8. b	13. b
4. c	9. a	14. a
5. a	10. d	15. d
16. d	21. c	26. a
17. d	22. b	27. d
18. c	23. d	28. a
19. b	24. c	29. b
20. a	25. d	30. d